returning to the original you

originalstrength
RESTORATION

tim anderson

FontLife Publications

Original Strength Restoration: Returning to the Original You
by Tim Anderson

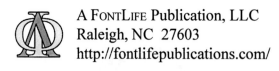

A FONTLIFE Publication, LLC
Raleigh, NC 27603
http://fontlifepublications.com/

Edition ISBNs:
Softcover: ISBN-10: 1-62422-022-3
           ISBN-13: 978-1-62422-022-7
Kindle: ISBN-10: 1-62422-023-1
           ISBN-13: 978-1-62422-023-4

First Edition 2014
Printed in the United States of America

Library of Congress Control Number: 2014947862

Original Cover Art by Danielle "Dani" Almeyda

Table of Contents

Special Thanks

I don't have enough words to express my gratitude and thanks to God for this amazing journey that is now called Original Strength. To know and see the lives that Original Strength has touched is nothing short of miraculous. Every day, I am left in awe. So, thank you, God!

Addie, thank you, too, for standing by my side. I don't know how you do all that you do, much less how you have the energy to deal with me. You are perfect, and I love you. Thank you.

Warning:

As always, you must get your physician's approval before beginning this exercise program. These recommendations are not medical guidelines but are for educational purposes only. You must consult your physician prior to starting this program or if you have any medical condition or injury that contraindicates physical activity. This program is designed for healthy individuals 18 years and older only.

See your physician before starting any exercise or nutrition program. If you are taking any medications, you must talk to your physician before starting any exercise program, including the *Original Strength* program. If you experience any lightheadedness, dizziness, or shortness of breath while exercising, stop the movement and consult a physician.

It is strongly recommended that have a complete physical examination if you are sedentary, if you have high cholesterol, high blood pressure, or diabetes, if you are overweight, or if you are over 30 years old, or if you are reading this. Please discuss all nutritional changes with your physician or a registered dietitian. If your physician recommends that you not use the *Original Strength Restoration* program, please follow your Doctor's orders.

All forms of exercise pose some inherent risks. The authors, editors, and publishers advise readers to take full responsibility for their safety and know their limits before practicing the exercises in this exercise program; and do not take risks beyond your level of experience, aptitude, training and fitness. The exercises and dietary programs in this program are not intended as a substitute for any exercise routine or treatment or dietary regimen that may have been prescribed by your physician.

The Original You

Do you remember when you were a child and you had an endless supply of energy? You could play hide-n-seek all day and never grow tired. You probably ran or skipped everywhere you went, just because you enjoyed it. Do you remember how just the thought of going to recess made it hard to concentrate on your schoolwork? What about your family gatherings? How often did you hear all your aunts and uncles say, "I sure wish I had that kind of energy" when you were growing up? Do you remember this?

Also, do you remember being able to eat anything you wanted and never gaining an ounce? Cookie dough, ice cream, pizza—you enjoyed it all. And never, not ever, did you worry about gaining weight, being fat, having high blood pressure, high cholesterol, or diabetes.

Chances are, when you were growing up, you moved a lot, you played a lot, you ate a lot of ridiculously good foods (at the time) and you laughed a lot. You had enough energy to supply a small town. You were filled with joy and laughter, and you ate conscience free.

When we were children, life was simple. We played hard, we ate hard, and we slept hard. When we were children, we were amazingly healthy—despite our poor food choices, or the dangerous games we used to play like dodge ball!

Think back, don't you remember these days of freedom? These days of "life"?

What if there were some things that we were never supposed to grow out of? What if we were always meant to have enough energy to power a locomotive? What if we were actually supposed to be able to eat any food, without fear or guilt? What if we were always supposed to have a positive body image, or no thought to a body image, because we always felt good?

Somewhere along the way, we have all settled for the notion that

7

children are childish and we should put away childish things once we become adults. Things like tooth fairies, unicorns, and superheroes are all supposed to be outgrown and we should learn to accept the reality that life is not all fun and games, or rainbows and roses. In truth, it is probably best that some things should be outgrown. Pacifiers look silly after about age two. But also in truth, not everything about a child's world is *childish*.

The problem with letting go of childhood, or dismissing most of the ways of a child, is that we end up letting go of a great deal of who we once were. We end up settling for some imagined notion that "Once you reach 30, everything starts to fall apart," or "I used to eat anything I wanted to and now if I just look at a doughnut, I gain 10 pounds," or "When I was I kid, I could run all day long and never get tired. I was the original Forest Gump. Now, I can barely catch my breath enough to walk to the mailbox."

Once upon a time, in land not so far away, you were strong, energetic, healthy, vibrant, joyful, and free. You were free from most of today's imagined and created fears about food, exercise, age, and illness. You were able to live a life full of excitement, adventure, and Kool-aid (sugar water).

Once upon a time, you LIVED!

What if the person you used to be, is still the person you were meant to be? What if you were never meant to trade your endless energy and appetite in for endless lethargy and lettuce wraps? What if being old, slow, tired, grumpy, and depressed is just a state of mind that we have settled for that stems from the lie that children are the way they are because they are children?

What would happen if we changed the way we think about the "cycle of life," if we refused to settle for aging and all of the endless "itises" that come with it? What would happen if we started to move again like we did when we were younger? What would happen if once we started moving again, we started letting go of our fears of food and the "lifestyle" prisons we put ourselves in? What if we just lived like we

8

once did? Like we were made to?

Yes, this is an absurd notion, unless you believe it is not. The mind is the most powerful thing in your body. Whatever you believe, whatever you settle for, is usually exactly what you will get.

Here's the truth: You were never meant to "grow up." Especially if growing up means getting slow, obese, lethargic, weak, fearful, depressed, apathetic and lifeless. None of us were meant for any of this. As children we all live the life we were created to until someone starts to tell us otherwise, until we "know better."

It is now time to "know better." We can return to the bodies we were meant to have, the bodies we once had. It all starts with the choice to believe we can. Once we have made this choice, we move—often and then more often. We move like we used to, and we enjoy it because we are starting to get younger again. Eventually, we even let go of our fears: food, germs, and spiders. Well, maybe not spiders.

What do you believe? Do you think the ways of a child are meant to be outgrown? Or do you believe we intuitively know exactly how to live, play, eat, and be as children (as "newer" people)? Do you believe you can become how you once were?

You can—if you choose to believe.

You can regain the Original You that you once were. In doing so, you can live the life that you were meant to live and make all your years golden.

The Broken Golden Years

Are you excited about living in the "Golden Years"? Are you already living in your Golden Years? Have you ever wondered why the later years in life are called the Golden Years, anyway? Look around you. Do you see anyone *living* in their Golden Years? Or, do the Golden Years that you see people existing in look more like the "Tarnished Years"?

If you really look around and you take notice of what is going on around you, you would see that many people are limping through life. The Golden Years in our lifetime now seems more appropriately aimed at people in their twenties.

Seriously. How many people do you know that concede, "after you turn thirty, everything just falls apart"? People are actually settling and **accepting** decline at age 30. It is even common practice to give, or get, black balloons and dead roses at the monumental 40th birthday. Yes, it is intended as a joke, but in my experience people most often joke about their own realities and beliefs.

Our modern world is full of broken people. By "broken," I mean that the world is full of people who are living lives that they were not meant to live. For example, in the United States it is now common to be labeled overweight or obese. It is also common, if not expected, for a person to use multiple medications to address the multiple issues that are now prevalent in our society, like high blood pressure, arthritis, depression, etc..

Speaking of medications, have you ever wondered why the list of side-effects for today's medications seem so much worse than the "ailment" they are intended for? Also, it should really go without saying that "If you experience blindness and loss of bladder control while taking Medication Z, please discontinue use and contact your doctor immediately." Do you ever wonder if people sit around thinking, "Well great, I can't see anymore, but at least my skin rash is gone. Wonder if I should tell my doctor..."?

Anyway, we have taken a wrong turn somewhere. We have learned how to convince ourselves that weakness and brokenness is a way of life. We have simply accepted too many lies.

Think of it. The Golden Years—a time that should be celebrated, a time where a man or a woman should rule and reign through the later parts of their lives with their heads held high, is now a time that is dreaded. If you mention the Golden Years today, assisted living homes and adult diapers probably come to mind more than images of long walks on the beach, or hiking through the hills. This is wrong.

Here is a truth that you should hold on to with all you've got: You came into this world full of life, and you are supposed to leave this world full of life. Being broken, weak and frail should be a rarity. It should never be the norm.

Your entire life should be full of strength and vitality. And, if at any point in life that you find yourself being less than full of life, you should fight and reclaim your vitality. Do not settle for the idea that you will wear out with age. Fight against that thought.

Why would it make sense for the best years of your life to be the first 20 to 30 years of your life? How much of "life" could you possibly experience or learn by the time you are 20? Or 30? Life is just getting started at age 30! By the way, did you know we are capable of living 120 years? 60 is supposed to be the midpoint! If anything, the last 60 years of your life should be approached the same way a child approaches the first years of his life: with wonder and excitement.

It's the truth. Have you ever looked at a child's face while he is exploring his world? What did you notice? What is the image in your mind's eye? Do you see a child whose eyes are full of life? There is a certain light, a joy, that emits from a child's eyes when he is exploring and growing through his world. A child's wonder filled eyes, his light filled eyes, are contagious. This light, this joy, is so strong that it makes you want to smile as well.

Children are often full of life, wonder, and joy. And you should be, too.

Whether you are 3, 33, or 133, you should have that same life and light emitting out of your eyes.

The point is, we came into this world with many gifts. Gifts that we were not meant to give away, or lose. The "You" that you were as a child is the "You" that you were made to be as an adult. The gifts inside of you, the gifts that made you "You," cannot be truly given away or truly lost. You can hide your gifts or put them up on a shelf, but they are always still inside of you somewhere.

What in the blue blazes am I talking about?

You can't give your health away, not entirely. And, you really can't lose your health either. You can, however, choose to put your health on a shelf and let it fade away. You can choose to let it decline. Even if you do though, you can find it, dust it back off and restore it. You cannot lose something that was put inside of you. For example, you were made to be strong. Because you were made to be strong, you can't really lose your strength. You can choose not to use it and walk in it, but you can't completely get rid of it. You were preprogrammed to be strong. The program that is inside of you can never be erased.

The reflexive strength you developed as a child was developed through a series of patterns and movements that were preprogrammed into you. The very same movements that developed your strength as a child are the very same movements that can redevelop or restore your strength as an adult, no matter what your age. The program—the operating system—for these foundational strength developing movements is still inside of you.

Does this make sense? You are wired to be strong. You can't really lose your strength. It is a gift. One you cannot give away. If you find yourself with less than the strength you were meant to have, with less than the strength you want to have, you can regain and restore your strength and your vitality.

You can regain your original strength. If you have your original strength, every stage and season of your life can be "golden." Owning your

12

original strength is owning your vitality. It allows you to be the "You" that you were created to be.

You should always be able to walk with a spring in your step. You should always be able to run through the woods like Daniel Day Lewis in *The Last of The Mohicans*. You should always have the light of life emitting from your eyes.

If you do not receive anything else from this book, receive this: You were meant to be healthy—ALWAYS! Do not settle for any idea, fact, notion or lie that tells you otherwise.

The Things We Leave Behind

When you were born, you were born mobile. In fact, you were more mobile than a sock monkey. Your body could bend and twist in almost any direction. You were pretty much a blank canvas waiting to reveal the beauty of movement, strength, grace, and power.

As you learned to move, you developed strength. Day in and day out you waged a war against gravity. Over time, you built a body that could withstand and endure the rigors of a wonderful game called Hide-n-Seek. This game ultimately embodied all athletic expressions know to man: sprinting, climbing trees, hurdling obstacles, tumbling at full speed and the occasional wrestling match. Do you remember that game?

There was also a time when you could sleep like a rock for 8 to 11 hours every night, and you would wake up every morning with a smile on your face. You would move—you would play—from the time you woke up until the time you went back to bed. Occasionally you would rest long enough to grab some food or maybe change the adventure you wanted to play in.

Speaking of food, do you remember when food was a freedom, a pleasure? When you were a child, you more than likely enjoyed good things to eat. You renewed and restored your body with food that tasted good. You ate whatever you wanted, whenever you wanted, and you were not condemned by it. You weren't imprisoned by it either. You didn't put yourself in a "food jail" by consuming your mind with macronutrient ratios, the timing of your meals, keeping food journals or counting calories. You simply enjoyed eating, and you were happy. You were free. You do remember this freedom, right?

We have left so many good things behind, in our past. Do you remember that place called "Outside"? Your parents used to always insist that you spent most of your time there. You probably insisted that you did, too. *Outside* was the ultimate playground. It is where you learned to run, climb, dig, build sand castles and forts, throw rocks, catch balls, and jump over creeks, or into mud puddles. *Outside* was that wonderful place, that "proving ground" where you developed your athletic ability and your problem solving intellect. It is the place where you discovered and satisfied your needs for exploration and adventure.

Outside was also a place that had those adventure-inspiring things called "swings." Remember those? When I was a kid, we used to try to swing as high as we could and then we would jump out at the top to see how far we could fly. We never cared about landing; we just wanted to fly. Did you ever do this? Do you have kids now? Do they ever get to experience flying like this?

The point is, once upon a time, you developed yourself: your strength, your emotions, your personality, your movements, and your thought processes through pure curiosity and a sense of adventure. There was a time in your life when curiosity literally moved you. It pulled you across a room; it begged you to climb a set of stairs. Have you ever noticed how most children cannot help but want to conquer a set of stairs, but most adults will do anything to avoid them? Isn't that funny?

The original you, the you that you once were, used to ignore the harsh word "NO!" and you relentlessly pursued climbing stairs as if there was a tractor beam pulling you up against all obstacles (your parents). You couldn't help it. You had to climb them. After all, you were made to explore. Your **curiosity** had no limits and it could not be contained.

Curiosity, foreign to many of us now, was once for us a whimsical sense of wonder that begged us to move with joy. Remember spinning in circles until you became dizzy and fell down? Did your parents yell at you to stop because they didn't want you to crack your head open? You still spun in circles anyway, with a giddy giggle and a smile on your face. How about practicing somersaults and flips? You probably used to do those almost every day, while smiling. These things used to fill you with joy. Today the thought of spinning in circles or flipping head over heals may actually fill you with dread.

What has happened? Who convinced us to put away these "childish" things that were once such a big part of who we were? How did we let our curiosity go? Why did we trade running, jumping and skipping for sitting and lounging? How did our thoughts change from, "I wonder if I can climb that tree…" to "Oh, that looks dangerous. I'll probably get hurt…"

We have left behind so many wonderful things. Things we were never supposed to leave behind. How did we do this? Why did we do this?

We stopped moving.

Movement—the one thing our bodies were made to do. The one thing that tied us together. It nourished our brains; it soothed our emotions. The very thing that made us who we were by supplying us with so many gifts: joy, wonder, imagination, resiliency, creativity, adventure and health. We gave it all away. We left all of these things behind. We lost ourselves—the bodies we were made to have—the day we stopped moving.

We haven't just lost ourselves either. We are losing our children, too. Many of us actually built the bodies we were meant to have as children, but today's child may never even get that far. Our world is now different. Playgrounds are dangerous. Outside is "boring." Hide-n-seek is not Angry Birds®. Today's child gets their sense of adventure from Nickelodeon®, iTunes®, Google Play® or Xbox®. Children today lack coordination, strength, posture and balance. If our future depends on our children, we need to make a change!

Today's child is getting robbed of so many of the gifts they were meant to have because we simply have too many distractions and too much information in our world today. That, and we've been paralyzed by fear. We are afraid of the risk of injury, and this fear is making us stupid. Please don't be offended. I actually saw on the news that one school had banned balls at recess because they might be used to throw at another child. If we don't get over ourselves and get over our fears, we are doomed to a life of existence—a black and white life that has no color, no joy, no adventure. This is not a life!

Fortunately, for all of us, we can regain everything that we have left behind and we can restore ourselves to the original individuals we were meant to be. Learning how to move again can return our strength, our joy, our creativity, our freedom and our lives. Yes, freedom can come from movement. Imagine a life where you can't move well, a life that is full of pain and mobility restrictions. Maybe this is where your body is today. If you can imagine this broken body, how much freedom do you imagine that this body has to enjoy life the way it was meant to? Do you think a tall flight of stairs would incite adventure or dread in this person? Would handrails be a necessity or a comfort? A person that moves well is a person that is free to move—free to run up stairs "just because"— free to engage in life without limits and constraints that are imposed on them by a body that has too many limits. Freedom is born from the ability to move. You were made move, and you were made to be free.

The good news is, as we touched on in the previous chapter, we cannot lose what we cannot give away. We all still have our movement template—our original operating system—programmed in our brains. This program still works. No matter how far away we might find ourselves from those first few years of life, our template for movement is still in us and we can activate it at anytime. And, if you are a parent of a child who may have missed out on the land of "Outside," or a child who cannot imagine a life without Wi-Fi, your child can still engage and activate this movement template and build the bodies they were meant to have as well. It is never too late and we are never too far gone.

This is really good news.

We can absolutely reclaim the gifts we've left behind and the person we were meant to be. All we have to do is start back at the beginning. Each of us has our own beginning. No matter where we are, we can start right there. Or, to say it another way, we can simply press reset.

Start Where You Are

Movement and life are like the game Monopoly®. We all start at the same place: we are born. We all have the same movement template—the same movement operating system—prewired in our bodies; and many of us develop in the same manner. However, after that starting place occurs, just like the wiles of Monopoly, life takes us on different journeys. None of us make it around the Monopoly board in the same manner. Some times we pass "Go" and collect 200 dollars. Sometimes we lose our turn because we are sitting in "Jail." The point is, once we are born, our lives take different paths.

Even though we all start out the same, few of us ever end up the same or have the same journey. Different events and circumstances in our lives give each of us a "different" body. And while we were all created to be healthy and strong, while we all share the same movement operating system, we may not all start back in the same place when it comes to restoring the body we were meant to have. We only start in the same place when we are born. After that, we can only begin our journey to restoration where our body will currently allow us to begin.

If this is confusing, think of it this way: Your body is different than mine in that you have a different history of movement and events in your body. If you and I were both going to start trying to restore our original bodies today, I may be able to start by crawling around like a baby, on my hands and knees, but you may not be able to. That could actually be too challenging for your body right now. You may actually have to start with a regression, a less challenging movement, than crawling. Within our original preprogrammed movement template, there are stages of progressions. Just as you have to crawl before you walk, you have to be able to lift your head before you crawl. Depending on how far away you have moved from your original strength, you may have to start closer to the beginnings of your original movement template when it comes to restoring and resetting your body.

We each simply have to start where we are. We can all restore our original strength, we just may not all start in the same place. That is good news! Your design is so wonderful, no matter where your body currently is, you can press reset and begin the process of restoration. It is easy, the program is already in you, you've already done it once, and you can do it again. You can absolutely restore yourself to the way you were meant to be. All you have to do is start where you are.

Pressing Reset Where You Are

In *Original Strength*, we introduce the five basic resets, the five basic original preprogrammed movements, that your body was designed to grow and develop from. These five movements are the foundation for life (movement, strength, health and vitality). Everything your body was meant to be able to do, everything your body was meant to be, comes from owning and maintaining this foundation. In fact, this original foundation of strength and life was intended to be maintained throughout your lifetime. Your body was designed to always and continually be "reset."

In other words, the design of the human body is so wonderful, that it is made to be self renewing. You were not made to break down with age or grow old and fall apart. The five original resets are actually designed to keep you tied together throughout your entire life. Yes, like a developing child, an adult should be moving and engaging in the resets, or their "adult progressions," on a daily, continual basis. For example, walking is a progression of crawling. Walking should be, is intended to be, a reset. However, for many people, walking is not a reset because they have "moved" too far away from their original, strong selves that they developed into as a child. They may have to restore walking by engaging in its regressions (crawling). But don't worry, if walking is not yet a reset for you, it soon will be.

In this section, we are going to look at the 5 major resets and explore their regressions. Remember, a regression is simply an easier, lower form of the reset. If a reset is too challenging for your body, then you need to regress that reset. You want to meet your body, to meet your movement foundation, where it is currently at. There is no need to try to run when you cannot walk well.

We are going to break each reset down so that no matter where your body is, no matter how far away you have moved from the you that you once were, you can begin the restoration process where you are now, today. These movements are simple, and your body already knows how to do them because they are "hard wired" into you. All we are doing when we press reset is helping your body to remember its original program design and dusting off all the wonderful connections in our nervous system. Once these wonderful connections are "dusted off," remembered, and restored, our foundation of strength and mobility are restored, thus allowing our bodies to become, again, what they were intended to be.

Yes, the simple ways of a child are the path to strength, mobility, freedom and life. Don't let this slip by you, *again.*

Please note: In *Original Strength: Regaining The Body You Were Meant To Have*, the reasoning behind the following 5 resets was covered in great depth. The following information about the 5 resets is not meant to be exhaustive, but supplemental to the information presented in *Original Strength*.

The Breath of Life

The first breath you ever took was a perfect, life giving breath. You inhaled through your nose, deep into your lungs, while using your diaphragm. Your diaphragm is your "breathing muscle," It is the muscle designed to pull air into the lower parts of your lungs, thus allowing you to fill your lungs completely and effortlessly. But breathing is not all the diaphragm is made to do. The diaphragm is also an integral part, if not the key, to solidifying your center. The diaphragm is perhaps the biggest secret to your strength. It works together with your pelvic floor, your transverse abdominis, and the muscles around your spine to form your inner core musculature.

It makes you solid and resilient from the inside out.

Without a properly functioning diaphragm, the body cannot produce as much force as it should be able to produce, nor can the body absorb and transfer force efficiently as it is made to do. Are you getting this? Breathing properly, with the diaphragm, is essentially core training. It is the original foundation for all of the strength, movement and ability that you were designed to have.

When it comes to understanding what the diaphragm does for your strength and resiliency, It may be helpful to think of the difference between a baseball and a whiffle ball. A baseball has a solid center. It is solid all the way through. You can hit a baseball with all of your might, hit a home run up into the stands, and the baseball retains its shape and structural integrity, You can use it and abuse it again and again. Now, look at a whiffle ball. A whiffle ball can have the same dimensions as a baseball, but the whiffle ball is hollow on the inside. It is not solid all the way through. You can hit a whiffle ball with all of your might, the same might you hit the baseball with, and the whiffle ball may not travel past second base. AND, more than likely, the whiffle ball will become damaged, cracked or dented. You cannot continually hit and abuse a whiffle ball in the same way you could a baseball because the whiffle ball does not have a solid center of structural integrity that can transfer the forces that are placed upon it. A whiffle ball is not resilient.

Our diaphragm, when we are using it properly, makes us more like the baseball; resilient and solid all the way through. When we are not using our diaphragm, we are more like the whiffle ball. We are not structurally sound and resilient; we can only take a few "hits."

But wait. If the diaphragm is the breathing muscle, how am I not using it when I breathe?

That's a great question. Many of us, through the stresses of life, or the pressures of self imposed value on aesthetics, have learned how to switch from using our diaphragm to breathe to using our "emergency muscles" to breathe. The muscles of our ribcage and our neck can also be used to pull air into our lungs. These muscles are to be reserved for breathing emergencies, for "fight or flight" situations. Yet somehow, due to the history of our own lives, many of us have learned how to make a switch and use these smaller, less efficient muscles to breathe instead of the intended primary breathing muscle, the diaphragm.

We have literally switched from using the preferred breathing method for the backup, emergency breathing method. And this is a big problem. Along with using the emergency breathing muscles to breathe comes other "emergency responses" from our body. These muscles are supposed to be reserved for fight or flight situations—situations that would require emergency responses—responses like increased adrenaline and increased cortisol. These are our fight or flight hormones. Again, hormones that are intended for emergencies. Living in a perpetual fight or flight state, continually breathing with our emergency muscles, causes huge hormonal imbalances by creating a constant state of stress throughout the body.

We are not supposed to live in a constant state of emergency. This creates a whole hosts of problems. Issues like adrenal fatigue, poor metabolism, acid reflux, high blood pressure, chronic fatigue, shortness of breath, anxiety, inflammation, weight gain, poor posture and so on, and on and on.

All of these issues could probably be mitigated if not eliminated through returning to the way we were designed to breathe, with our diaphragm.

This is vitally important to restoring your health, to restoring yourself to the way you were meant to be.

Breathing properly is the ONE thing that makes you resilient and capable of living a life of vitality. To say that breath is life is completely true, but for so many more reasons than just to inhale oxygen. It is your breath that solidifies you and makes you resilient. It is your breath that allows you "rest and digest," to be set free from the stresses of life.

Life starts and ends with breath. And it is here that we return to our most important reset: Breathing, the way we were designed to breathe, by using our diaphragm.

Breathing

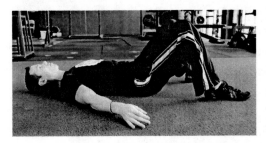

Here is a simple, easy position to start remembering how to use your diaphragm. Simply lie down, bend your knees, rest your feet on the floor, place your tongue on the roof of your mouth and **breathe in and out of your nose**.

Try to pull the air you are breathing in, all the way down into your feet—use your imagination and breathe deep.

If done right, the belly should rise as you breathe in, and fall as you breathe out.

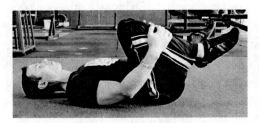 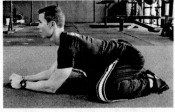

Sometimes, it is easier to find your diaphragm if you get "shorter." In these two positions above, I have made my body shorter. These "short"

23

positions provide more information for the brain, as the belly will expand against the thighs. This makes it easier for the brain to find and use the diaphragm as there is more sensory information surrounding the diaphragm and the pelvic floor. These short positions also "wake up" the pelvic floor and bring it closer to the diaphragm. Remember, the diaphragm and the pelvic floor work together to form your inner core—they make your center solid!

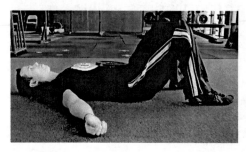 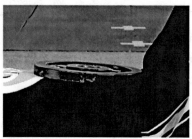

Sometimes, still, we may need a little more feedback, or information, to help us find our diaphragm. Here, in these pictures, I have placed a 10-pound weight plate on my belly. The plate will provide awareness of my belly to my brain, and perhaps help me more easily locate my diaphragm as I breathe. The goal for me is to make the plate rise and fall with my breath. If you try this idea, you do not need to use 10-pound weight plate! A shoe, or any object will work just fine for you.

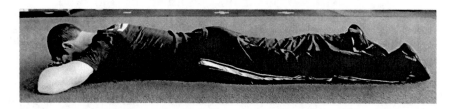

This position is known as "crocodile breathing." This is another great way to locate your diaphragm. Here, your belly pushes against the floor as your breathe in and your low back rises. If you are breathing in your chest while in this position, the floor will give you feedback for that as well. You want to be able to breathe deep, all the way down to your feet. Done properly, this not only helps you find and use your diaphragm, but it feels amazing and it can really help melt your stress away.

More Positions

These are but a few positions of potentially infinite positions. The positions listed here do make it relatively easy to find and remember how to use your diaphragm. Ideally, you want to be able to always breathe using your diaphragm no matter what position, or situation, you find yourself in.

If you spend enough time practicing and remembering how to use your diaphragm you will eventually find that you no longer need to practice. One day you will discover that you are simply breathing the way you were designed to breathe; whether driving, walking, running, working or sleeping, you will be using your diaphragm. Along with that, along with restoring your natural breathing pattern, you will also find that you have less stress in your life, more energy, more mobility and more strength. You will be healthy.

WARNING:

This is the one reset you will be most tempted to skip. Do not make this mistake. This is the most critical reset of all. This is the first place to start on the road to restoration!

It is Okay To Nod Off

Your vestibular system (your balance system) is probably the most important sensory system in your body. Truly, every system you have is *the most important system* in your body because if you are lacking one system, your body will not be whole and complete as it should be. However, the vestibular system deserves extra special recognition as the other sensory systems like the visual system and the proprioceptive system are routed into and through your vestibular system.[1] In short, your vestibular system is the foundation of your sensory systems. It is also the foundation of who you are.

Did you know that four months before you ever see the light of the world, four months before your eyes ever see day light and before your lungs ever breathe air, your vestibular system is completely, fully functioning and operational?[2] Four months before you are born your vestibular system is receiving information and nourishing and knitting your brain together. Every time your mother sneezed, coughed or laughed she stimulated your vestibular system and this stimulation was used to develop your brain. When your mother took walks, the rhythm of her gait actually nourished your brain and helped develop your body because it was feeding your vestibular system with the wonderful rhythm of her movement.

After you were born, a new force other than your mother, gravity, stimulated your vestibular system. Once your body realized the true pull of gravity in the "outside world," your vestibular system started working on its new job: getting and keeping your head level with the horizon. We were all preprogrammed with a self-righting reflex—one of the main roles of our balance system is to keep our heads up so we can see the world. It is this reflex that helps govern how capable we can become because our bodies are designed to follow our heads. Our brains adjust our posture and position in order to keep our heads level with the horizon. But before I get into that, consider this:

You are essentially a product of the information your vestibular system receives.

Your vestibular system lives in your head, behind your ears, and it is connected to every single muscle in your body.[3] It governs how well you are reflexively "wired" together. Your posture, your balance and your reflexive strength are all determined by how nourished, or malnourished, your vestibular system is. Pay attention here: moving your head reflexively affects all the muscles in your body, especially your postural muscles. Your balance, posture and coordination are all built and determined by how well you move your head.[4]

The key to strength and health lies in our ability to move our heads. Our entire body is reflexively wired to the little movement sensors (the vestibular system) that lives in our head—a head that sits on top of a neck that is capable of full flexion, extension and rotation. In other words, our head is made to be moved in almost every way imaginable. It is this movement that activates the vestibular system, which in turn provides reflexive and anticipatory strength, stability and movement when and where it is needed.

What?

The ability to move your head freely, enables you to have a body that has a foundation of strength. The kind of strength that prevents you from getting injured should you slip and fall. The kind of strength that allows you to engage in any physical activity without the fear of getting injured. Your reflexive strength, which is determined by the health of your vestibular system, is the strength that preserves you. It should also be noted that the better you can move your head, the better your righting reflex can accurately and reflexively adjust all the muscles in your body in order to keep your head level with the horizon. Again, the body is made to follow the head, quickly and reflexively. You could even say that the body is made to follow the head before the head even moves, in anticipation of the head moving.

So, clearly our design shows that we are made to move our heads and that this movement nourishes and preserves us. But what happens if we don't move our heads? The exact opposite. Moving our heads "sharpens" our reflexes. Not moving our heads "dulls" our reflexes. If all the muscles in our body are tied to our ability to move our heads, then not moving our heads, in a sense, unties all of our muscles, and our reflexes become dull. We lose our reflexive strength, our foundation of strength and health. Our ability to move quickly in order to avoid injury is diminished. Our would-be anticipatory actions become *after the incident* reactions—they become too little, too late.

You have heard this all of your life: Use it or lose it. And most of us have lost it—our reflexive strength, that is. However, we still have our vestibular systems and we still have the same design that the vestibular system was meant to function with. In other words, we can regain our reflexive strength by relearning how to move our heads again.

We can actually nod our way back to health. That is awesome! Wouldn't you agree? (Nod your head for "YES!")

Head Control Positions

Rotation

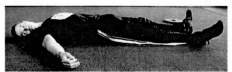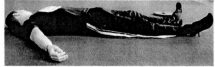

Here is a great place to start when it comes to regaining head control. Simply rest your head on the floor, place your tongue on the roof of your mouth, and rotate your head from side to side as far as it will comfortably go. Do not force your head to go where it does not want to go, and do not move into pain! Simply move where your body will let you go. **Lead with your eyes!!!!**

Flexion

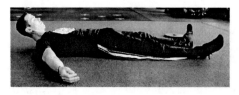

This is neck flexion. Flexing the neck activates your abdominal muscles—at least it should! Start with your head on the floor, place your tongue on the roof of your mouth and tuck your chin to your chest. Notice how your abdominals contract! This is reflexive core training! This is strength!

Flexion and Rotation

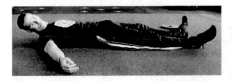 Can you do both? Once you get good at rotating your head and flexing your head while lying on your back, try performing both at the same time. Regaining the ability to control your head will allow you to regain the ability to control your body!

Extension (We call these head nods!)

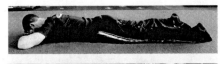
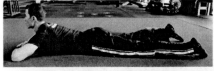 Your ability to raise your head into extension is a key to health. Raising your head strengthens your back and spinal postural muscles. Just as flexing your neck is tied to your abdominals, extending your neck is tied to your back muscles.

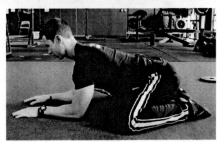 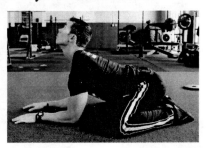

Flexion and Extension (More Head Nods!)

When not lying on the belly, you can practice head nods by moving into both flexion and extension. Head nods, can also be a great way to mobilize the spine and restore "good" reflexive posture. Truly, in this position, you could practice flexion, rotation, and extension—and you should!

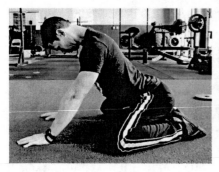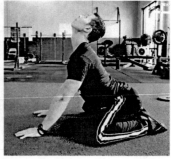

Extend your head up as far as it will let you go. If you can see the ceiling, look to the sky! If not, don't sweat it. Eventually, you just might be able to.

Extension and Rotation

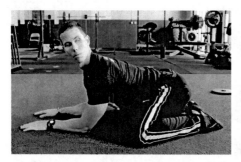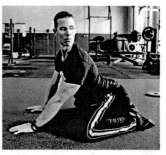

Can you hold your head up and rotate? Try to look at your own feet, or your own "backside."

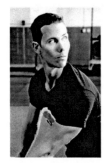 Don't forget, lead with your eyes. The eyes lead, then the head, then the body.

Where the head goes, the body will follow. If your head isn't going anywhere, where are you going to be able to go? Mastering head control is a key to being strong and resilient throughout your entire life, it is a key to restoring the body you were meant to have.

Silly Rabbit, Rolling Is For Kids!

The very first time you discovered you could roll over, you found something that you would idealize forever: Freedom. When you learned how to roll across the floor of your home as a child, you learned how to go places. You learned how to manipulate your body enough to get where you wanted to go. And in doing so, you found a freedom that ran along side of your curiosity. This was a powerful combination that allowed you, and begged you, to keep moving and exploring your way to true health and resiliency. There is no freedom like the freedom to go where you want to go and to be able to explore the places you want to explore. Just ask any 16 year-old when they first get their license!

Rolling was your first "vehicle" or mode of transportation from one spot to another. Even if that spot was only 4 inches away from where you started, it was enough for you to learn how to make it 4 feet, and then 4 yards. I remember when my first son, Luke, learned how to roll. He rolled all over the house. He could get anywhere he wanted to go by simply rolling all over the floor. I thought I was going to have to tie a bell to him because he was rolling like a ninja!

Ninja skills aside, rolling is also where you first started tying your opposite hips to your opposite shoulders, connecting them. When you learned to roll, you reflexively connected your entire body through your center, your "X" (The body is one big X), and in doing so, you continued to lay a bombproof foundation of strength. Not only did you connect your center by getting your hips and shoulders tied together, but you also further sharpened all of your postural reflexes and enhanced your balance because you activated your vestibular system with every roll that you made.

Rolling, like moving the head, activates the vestibular system. In fact, it is through head movement and the righting reflex that we really learn the ability to roll. Developmentally, you continued to build on the strength and movement foundations that you laid with each new movement discovery. In other words, the strength you built from learning how to control your head, is the strength that enabled you to learn how to roll—

more than likely, but perhaps not for everyone. Then, the strength you developed from learning how to roll, became the strength that enabled you to learn how to creep.

But let's roll on.

Rolling is also an extremely sensory rich movement that floods your brain with nourishment. This is because rolling stimulates your largest proprioceptive organ, your skin. The proprioceptive information, the information and sensations received from your skin and your muscles, is routed on top of and through your vestibular system. Those two sensory systems work together, along with your visual system, to feed your brain with a flood of information. Information that not only continues to sharpen your reflexes, but it also paints a rich picture, or map, of where your body is and what it is doing. In other words, your vestibular system and your proprioceptive system work together to fine tune all of your movements, even the movements that you don't notice—the ones that enable your balance, posture and coordination.

Again, rolling is where we really start tying our bodies together. It is where we start becoming fully integrated: Body parts to body parts, muscles to brain, sensory systems to sensory systems. Rolling makes us one. If you have discovered that your body is no longer one with itself, it could be time to roll yourself back together.

Segmental Rolling

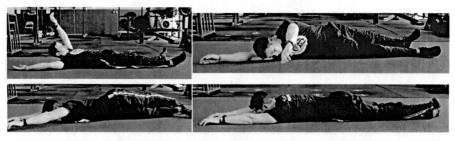

Segmental rolling is done by using either a leg, or the head and an arm, to roll from your back to your belly, or to roll from your belly to your back. Segmental rolling should ultimately be fluid, like a beautiful ocean wave rolling over from one side to the other.

This is a segmental roll from the back to the belly using the left arm and the head. In segmental rolling, the body should roll over segment by segment.

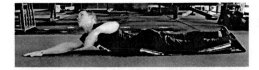

Here, in this segmental roll from the belly to the back, the head leads the show. The torso follows, then the pelvis, then the hips.

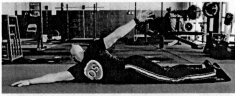

Remember, whether rolling with the legs (not shown), or the head and arms, the body should flow over piece by piece.

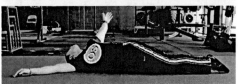

Egg Rolls

For some people, learning how to roll with fluidity can be a challenge if not aggravating. Some people roll over like a log; they have no fluidity. Other people may not be able to roll over at all.

If this is you, do not fret. When you were a child you didn't roll over perfectly on your first try. In fact, I am pretty sure the first time you rolled over was an accident. The point is that you probably explored and accidentally found out how to roll segmentally through rolling anyway your head and body would allow you to go. You may have even done something like the egg roll.

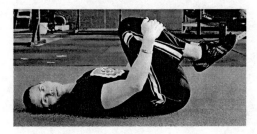

Do you remember this breathing position?

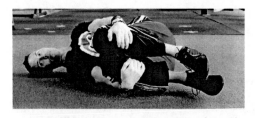

Simply lie on your back, fold your knees towards your chest and hold them. Now, look right and roll to the right.

Lead with your eyes.

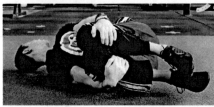 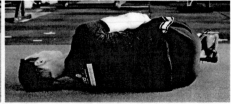

Next, look left, and roll your body to the left. It is okay if you have to help out with your elbows to roll back over. Eventually, you will not have to. Notice that the egg roll initiates rolling with the head rotating from side to side. Rolling builds off of head control. Learn how to move your head, learn how to roll your body.

Half Rolls and Reaches

Some people cannot roll simply because they are trying to think their way through rolling and they have forgotten why the learned how to roll in the first place: they were trying to get something. Babies learn how to roll because their curiosity begs them to investigate their world. Babies find a target, and then they go get it. As adults, sometimes we just need a target to reach for. You can remember how to roll simply by reaching for something you want.

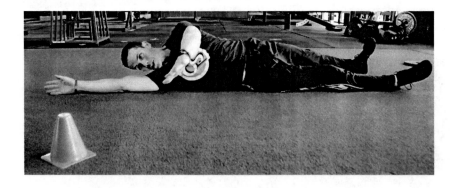

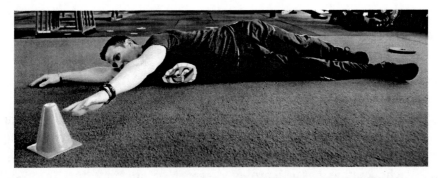

The act of reaching for something can help you remember how to roll. Place an object near you, but out of your reach, and reach for it. If you are reaching with your arms, relax your lower body. If you are reaching with your legs, relax your upper body. Simply reach and allow your reach to roll you over. Reach as far as you can without tensing up. If you tense up, return to where you started and try again.

Have fun with reaching and place the object in several not so easy places to get to. Place it over your head, behind you, beside your legs towards your feet, place it wherever you want. Just be creative and let your reach "teach" your roll.

The Wisdom of The Rocking Chair

We have somehow known for centuries that rocking soothes. How do we try to calm an upset child? We sway, or rock him. How do we try to get our babies to fall asleep? We sit and rock them in a rocking chair. Intuitively, we have always known that there is something very calming about rocking. Children know this, too. Have you ever seen an upset child who maybe has a learning disorder or an emotional disorder? What do they do to calm themselves and cope? They rock.

Rocking is every bit of an emotional reset as it is a physical one. Combined with diaphragmatic breathing, rocking cannot only restore you, but it can soothe you. Rocking can literally help the stress of your day melt away. But rocking also does much more than that; it soothes the stresses in your body as well. Rocking is one of the "Big Bang" resets because it integrates all the major joints of the body and it continues to further make the body one cohesive movement canvas, from which you could paint any movement imaginable.

Rocking mobilizes the ankles, knees, hips, spine, shoulder, neck, elbows and wrists. Each rhythmic movement of rocking takes all of these separate joints and unifies them together, as one, along with all the muscles and tendons that surround each of these joints. Each rhythmic forward-and-back motion unifies you. Rocking prepares you for graceful, flowing, movement. Movement without hitches, movement without pain, and movement without limitations.

Perhaps one of the most powerful things about rocking is that being on all fours, being on your hands and knees with your head held up, reflexively tunes all of your muscles, especially your postural muscles. Posture, good or bad, is a reflex. It is a position you have, not a position you strive to hold. Rocking is what sets your posture as a child and it can restore your posture as an adult. If you want good posture, you need to be reflexively "on." Rocking turns you "on" and resets both your body and your mind.

The Standard Rocking Position

Rocking should look like this:

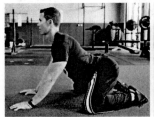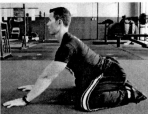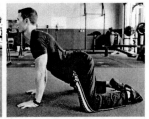

Simply get down on the floor, on your hands and knees, and rock back and forth. Keep your head and chest "up." Your head should always be held up when rocking.

Rocking should not look like this:

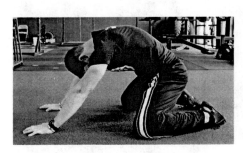

When rocking, we do not want to lose the natural curves of our spine (look at above pictures). The back should not round and the head should not drop.

Only rock back as far as you can WHILE maintaining the good posture of your spine. If your spine starts to round or your head starts to drop, you have gone far enough.

When you have reached the end of your range of motion, the point where you can still maintain your spine, practice the resets of breathing and head nods. These 2 resets can help open up your hips and restore your reflexive stability.

Eventually, as your reflexive stability is restored, you will be able to rock further back while maintaining the natural postural curves of your spine.

This is the standard foot position for rocking:

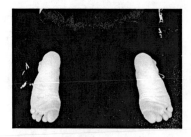

In the standard rocking position, the feet should be held in plantar flexion and relatively neutral. That is, the tops of your feet should be touching the floor.

Foot Position Matters

Your feet were made to move. There are 26 bones and 33 joints in your feet.[5] These joints were made for movement. Rocking in, and with, different foot positions is a great way to restore and mobilize the feet and ankles. If you can restore your feet and ankles, you can restore your body!

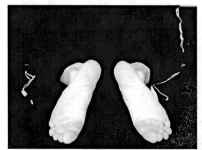
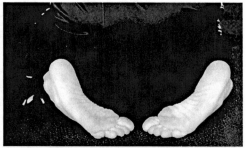

Plantar flexion, heals in   **Plantar flexion, heals out**

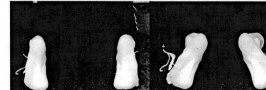
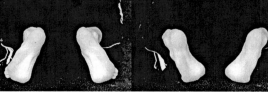

Dorsiflexion   Dorsiflexion, heals in   Dorsiflexion, heals out
neutral position

Ideally, you want to be able to rock with your feet in any of these positions. Your feet however, may have a different idea. It is okay if your feet do not want to move easily into these positions. You may simply have to encourage them and be patient with them. You also may have to help them out by isolating one foot with another foot.

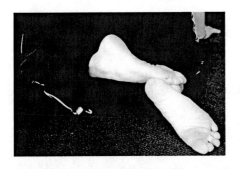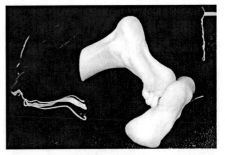

Here are two examples of how you can use one foot to help get the other foot into the position you want to rock in. After you rock mobilizing the one foot, you can switch and mobilize the other foot.

If you have stiff, immobile feet, you may experience cramping when trying to get your feet in some of these positions. Eventually, this will pass and your feet will become more mobile.

One Leg At a Time

Sometimes, the feet just need a little more attention. This is a variation of rocking on one leg at a time. In this position, the position that many kids naturally sit in on the floor, it is a bit easier to mobilize the feet and ankles. When rocking in this sitting position, keep your head up and chest tall, but don't focus on the spine like we teach in the standard rocking position. This form of rocking here is focused mainly on the feet, and ankles, and knees, and hips… If you keep your chest up, the spine will take care of itself.

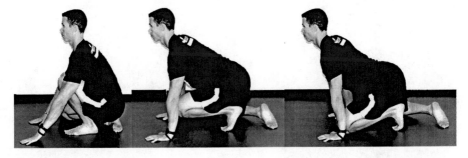

Start as close to this first position as possible (you could do this once!)— one foot is underneath and behind you, and the bottom of the front foot is in full contact with the floor. Then shift your weight forward as though you are about to crawl. Allow your foot, knee, and hip to move as far as they will let you take them. Then, rock back to the stating position. You can play with angles here. In the above pictures, my knee is inside of my elbows and underneath my chest. You can also let the knee rock outside the elbows, placing more emphasis on the outer part of the foot.

Note: Both feet get mobilized in this position. One is mobilized in dorsiflexion and the other is mobilized in plantar flexion. Switch this position to work both sides evenly. Rocking in this manner can really help wake up and restore the feet and ankles. It also simply feels good.

Remember, if you find it difficult to get into one of the above foot positions, simply go where your body will let you go. For example, if you are trying to get on the balls of your feet (the dorsiflex position) but you are barely able to get on your toes, that is okay. Rock where your feet will allow you to go. Restoration of the foot and ankle can take a little time. Just be patient and play with the positions above; especially the positions that are the hardest to get into!

Rocking can help restore you: physically, mentally, and emotionally. It is complete and whole integration. It sets your posture, it mobilizes most of your joints, it sharpens your reflexes, it soothes your emotions, and it steadies your thoughts.

Rock yourself back to the original you.

Crawling is Walking

We were made to stand, walk, and run on two feet. Walking is our primary contra-lateral gait pattern. At least it is supposed to be, contra-lateral that is. There are many people walking around today who are not really "walking." Walking is supposed to be a very graceful, fluid and even powerful contra-lateral gait pattern (opposite limbs are supposed to deliberately and rhythmically move in coordination with one another). Because walking is to be a contra-lateral gait pattern, it would require both hemispheres of the brain to be in constant communication with themselves and it would also reflexively continue to keep the body tied together. The deliberate motion of the shoulders working with the hips keeps the body connected; it keeps your center solid. From this design, it is easy to see that walking is supposed to be the "exercise" that keeps us renewed and restored. Walking should be our giant reset button! But for many of us, it is not.

Many of us have forgotten, or unlearned, that walking is to be a contra-lateral gait pattern. Many of us today actually walk around without using our shoulders at all. Our arms just hang motionless, or we keep them in our pockets, or we use them as podiums for our phones. We walk, but we are not walking in the movement of our intended design. We are not renewing ourselves with every step. But we should be. Every step we take should be a reset. That is how we were designed.

For many of us, we simply need to reprogram and restore our walk back to its intended design. The way we do this is the way we did it the first time: we crawl. Crawling is the original contra-lateral gait pattern off of which walking is supposed to be built. Crawling is "walking" on all fours.

This very deliberate coordinated contra-lateral pattern is the pattern that finished tying you together as a child. This is the pattern that was intended to establish your foundation of reflexive strength. It is like the Super Glue® that literally took all your parts and combined them to make you one fluid movement mosaic. Crawling finished integrating all of your sensory systems into one big sensory system—YOU.

41

Your auditory system, visual system, proprioceptive system and your vestibular system were all combined together through crawling. I know, I left out sense of smell. I believe it probably integrated your sense of smell, too, but I've never read anything to say that it did.

Crawling also finished integrating your nervous system to your muscular system. It established your reflexive strength. It began building your balance. It coordinated your hands to your eyes and your eyes to your head. It further set your posture; and it established your gait pattern. Or, at least it was supposed to. If you skipped crawling, however, you may have skipped over a few of these wonderful, benefits. Don't fret if this is you, the crawling program is still in you!

Even if you did not skip crawling, you may have lost many of its wonderful benefits if you have spent the last 40 years of your life being sedentary. For many of us, we just need to go back to the beginning to reclaim the things we have given up. Thankfully, as I said, the crawling program is still in us no matter what age or stage in life that we find ourselves in. We can press reset with crawling and we can regain the strength, health and life that we were designed to have. We can once again regain our automatic reset, walking, and restore our bodies with every step that we take. In doing so, we can "walk" through this life as participants and conquerors instead of defeated spectators.

Believe it or not, not everyone can crawl well. In fact, some people may need to begin with crawling regressions.

All of that to say, let's learn how to crawl!

The Standard for Crawling

Crawling should look like this:

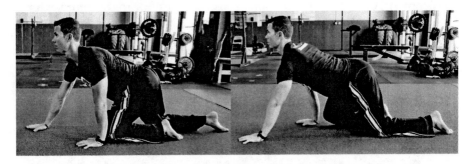

Notice that the head is up and the spine has the same good posture that we discussed in the rocking section. Crawling is a contra-lateral movement—opposite limbs should move together in coordination with one another. Also notice that the feet drag along the floor and the knees track inside the elbows, underneath the body.

Crawling should not look like this:

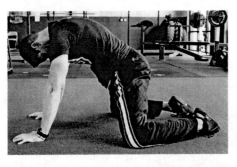

Crawling like this displays a lack of reflexive strength. The good spine posture has been lost and the back is now in flexion. Also, the head is down displaying lack of head control, or fear that the floor will soon disappear.

Warning: If the head is held down when you crawl, you may run into something! Keep your head up so you can see where you are going!

If your crawl looks similar to the above picture, you may need to take a step back and work on some crawling regressions. Don't worry, these regressions are still "resets" and they will help restore your body.

Dead Bugs

Dead bugs are a great way to reflexively strengthen the abdominals, the front of your "X" (your body), as well as improve contra-lateral limb coordination. They yield many of the same wonderful benefits as crawling and they help build the reflexive strength that is needed to crawl well.

This is what dead bugs look like:

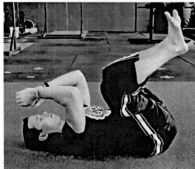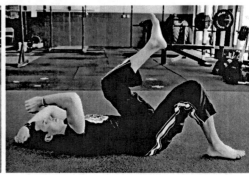

Start with all four of your limbs in the air. Keep your knees pulled up towards your chest so that your tail bone is off the floor. From here, you are going to lower your opposite limbs together and then bring them back to the starting point together. Alternate from side to side. Can you do 50 reps?

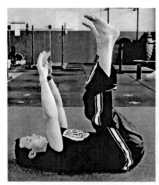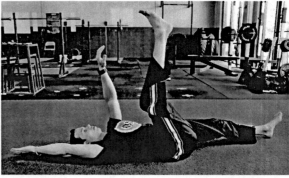

As your strength builds, or if it is easy to do with your elbows and knees bent, you can straighten them and place more demand on your abdominals. Be sure to keep the knee pulled up towards the chest with the leg that remains in the air. If you can perform 50 reps of these, while keeping your tail bone off the floor, you are on your way to crawling!

Birddogs

Dead bugs reflexively strengthen the front of your X, and bird dogs reflexively strengthen the back of your X, along with improving contralateral limb coordination. These too, make a great regression for building the strength and coordination needed for crawling.

This is what a birddog looks like:

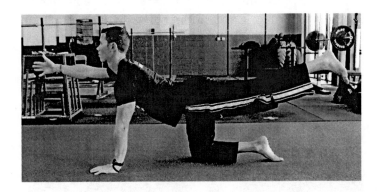

To begin, start on your hands and knees, as if you were about to start crawling. Then, lift your opposite arm and leg away from each other. Notice that the head is held "up," This is a coordinated, contra-lateral movement that yields many of the same benefits that crawling does.

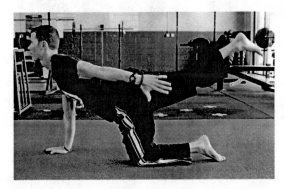

Here is another variation of the bird dog that is more inline with our true gait pattern. In this variation, the opposite limbs move in the same direction, just as they do when you walk.

Ideally, you want to be able to perform these birddog examples from side to side with ease. And, eventually, you want to be stable while performing the birddogs. If you can do these and dead bugs easily, you should be ready to crawl!

Cross-crawls

Cross-crawls are technically not a regression to crawling. However, they are included here because anyone, regardless of their ability, or physical condition, can participate in cross-crawls. You may have wrist issues, knee issues, or fear issues about being down on the floor, but you can still perform cross-crawls no matter what your issues are.

Cross-crawls are the most accessible, and potentially most powerful reset. DO NOT underestimate them. Their simplicity can be life changing.

Cross-crawl Variations:

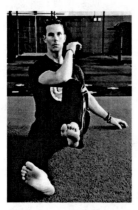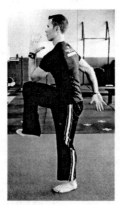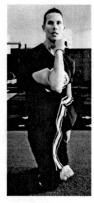

Cross-crawls are performed by simply touching your opposite arm to your opposite leg. If you have the mobility it can be your opposite elbow to your opposite knee, your opposite hand to your opposite foot, or even just your finger tips to your thigh. As long as your arm crosses the midline of your body and touches any part of your opposite leg, that is a cross-crawl.

They can be done standing up, lying down, in a chair, a wheel chair, or a waterbed. Anyone, with any condition, in any location, in any situation, can perform cross-crawls. This simple move can restore mental function, physical balance, mobility, strength, and hope. Again, DO NOT dismiss this simple, restorative movement.

The Power of the Tongue

This Chapter may look somewhat familiar if you are one of those who received The Missing Chapter from *Original Strength*. This is a chapter we offered to the readers of that book after it was published. It is valuable, so I am including it here:

> *Death and Life are in the power of the tongue, and those who love it will eat its fruit.—Proverbs 18:21*

This is true on so many different levels. The tongue is perhaps one of the most powerful muscles in the human body; not just because it can form words that can build up or tear down, but because it can be used to build a reflexively strong and capable body. The tongue can make you unstoppable. Or, it can pull you apart.

Have you ever heard the phrase "You will have what you say?" Your words matter. The words you speak generally come from your inner most thoughts—your beliefs. If your thoughts are riddled with fears and doubts, your words will express these thoughts and you will create weaknesses in your body and your life. Saying things like, "I can't," "I have to be careful, I don't want to hurt my back again," "I'm afraid I might get hurt," or even "I'm too old," will produce exactly what you say. Speaking negativity will result in negative consequences. These kind of words will tear you down and keep you from living a life of vitality.

However, thoughts and words of strength and health will also produce a life filled with strength and health. If you believe and know that you are resilient, you will be resilient. If you start saying things like, "I can do this," or "I am strong," or "I am not afraid," you will start to unlock your body's potential.

This might seem odd, but your words are seeds. The seeds you plant today will grow and become what you will have tomorrow. Your words build your beliefs, your beliefs actually change the shape of your brain— neural pathways in your brain actually represent them, especially if you say and think the same thoughts over and over again.[6] Eventually, these thoughts, these neural pathways effect your emotions and your physical health.

Don't believe me? Consider this: One man can be told he is going to die in one month from a certain disease. He can believe what he is told, start telling others, start imagining his last days, and sure enough he does die in about one month. Another man can be told that he is also going to die in one month from the exact same disease. This man, however, can choose to not believe what the doctor says. He can start to tell people, I am NOT going to die. I AM GOING to live. He can resist and fight the thoughts of death and depression, and sure enough he can live and boggle the minds of his doctors.

Stories like this happen all the time. What is the difference? Words. Your words and the words you listen to from others are seeds. How you sow them and cultivate them shape your outcome. You need to be mindful of the words you say and the thoughts that you keep. You need to watch your tongue!

The Sixth Reset

The power of the tongue does not stop with words though. The tongue itself plays a critical role in your reflexive strength. The natural resting position of the tongue is on the roof of your mouth, right behind your front teeth. This position is actually a reset for the body.

We have already discussed the benefit of diaphragmatic breathing: it is crucial for tying your body together and developing reflexive strength. Placing the tongue on the roof of the mouth encourages nasal breathing, thus encouraging diaphragmatic breathing. You can breathe diaphragmatically through your mouth or through your nose, but we are supposed to naturally breathe through our noses. There is a strength benefit to doing so. The nasal passages are smaller than the opening of the mouth. Breathing in through the narrow nasal passages actually helps create more inter-abdominal pressure between your diaphragm and your pelvic floor. That is to say that nasal breathing helps your center become stronger and more resilient by creating a "muscle girdle." The tongue

49

encourages "reflexive breathing strength."

The tongue also has a great effect on the vestibular system. Placing the tongue on the roof of the mouth stimulates the tongue ligaments that are connected to the vestibular system.[7] Remember, the vestibular system is connected to every single muscle in your body! Also, because the tongue stimulates the vestibular system, it also activates the RAS (the Reticular Activating System), which increases focus and balance.[8] The RAS is responsible for regulating arousal and sleep-wake transitions in people. The tongue can stimulate the RAS system and make you more alert and able to focus, kind of like a "wake up" call or a cup of coffee. It's a mental alertness reset! The more alert the brain is, the faster the body's reflexes can react.

Resting the tongue on the roof of the mouth also allows the neck to move through a full range of motion and can even improve your posture. Try this: Lie on the floor, on your back. Let your tongue rest on the bottom of your mouth and perform a few neck raises. Now place your tongue on the roof of your mouth and perform a few more neck raises. Did you notice how much easier and further you could raise your neck? Remember, the movement of the head and neck stimulates the vestibular system. By holding your tongue in its natural resting position, you allow your neck to move through a full range of motion (you may even gain a full range of motion that you haven't had in quite a while). Moving your neck through a full range of motion, further stimulates your vestibular system and effects every single muscle in your body, especially the muscles of the core!

Another fascinating tip about the tongue is that placing the tongue on the roof of your mouth and then pressing it hard, applying pressure, can also stimulate the nerves and relax the facial muscles around the eyes, ears and mouth. This can improve nerve and muscle function of the eyes, facial muscles and mouth.[9] The tongue is intimately tied to your body's reflexes.

Here is a reminder from the Vestibular System Chapter in *Original Strength*:

50

Mastering head control is essential to balance, posture and coordination, therefore mastering head control is essential for strength and vitality. The tongue plays no small role in mastering head control! The tongue helps facilitate head control and its placement has a direct effect on balance and posture as the tongue activates the vestibular system. This is HUGE! Controlling your tongue is key to having a strong, healthy body! Marinate on this. Something as simple as placing your tongue on the roof of your mouth can help you build a reflexively strong body.

Placing your tongue where it belongs is a reset. Remembering and learning how to keep it there will restore you. It is really quite an amazing and powerful muscle. It can articulate words that yield the fruit of its seeds; and it can reset, restore and preserve the health of the body.

Why not take all the brakes off your body? Start being mindful of the words that you say and start being mindful where you allow your tongue to rest. If you get riddled with fear, start speaking boldness. Speak life. Speak words of life until you believe them! And, when you are performing your resets (rolling, rocking, head nodding, crawling), or any activity for that matter, place your tongue on the roof of your mouth, breathe through your nostrils and "super charge" your reflexive strength.

The truth is, your tongue controls everything about you. If you learn how to control your tongue you can build the foundation, the original strength that you were truly meant to have. This is not just a physical foundation either; this is a foundation that extends way beyond physical health. Remember, death and life are in the power of the tongue. Choose life!

The Resets Within The Resets

Now that we've learned about the power of the tongue, it might be a good time to discuss the resets within the resets. There are 3 resets that can actually make the other resets work better. To say it another way, there are 3 resets that are foundational before the other resets can be true resets:

- Tongue position
- Breathing with the diaphragm
- Head Nods (mastering head control)

Without these 3 resets, the other resets will not have as big of an impact as they should. The truth is, these three resets should be automatically and continuously maintained at all times. They should always be "running in the background." No, we shouldn't be performing head nods constantly, but we should be using our heads, turning our neck, and exercising head control throughout our days. But yes, we should be breathing with our diaphragm with every breath we take, unless we are in danger; and we should keep our tongue rested on the roof of our mouth, unless we are speaking.

These 3 resets should be our natural default. They are intended to be maintained without conscious thought. And they can be if they are not, with a little conscious effort. We can get to the point in our lives where we no longer have to consciously breathe with our diaphragm and we no longer have to consciously keep our tongue on the roof of our mouth. We can get to the point where it is completely natural to turn our heads in every direction our necks were made to move, on purpose, out of desire to move and see what's going on around us.

We can get "there." "There" is where we used to be. And "there" is still there. Waiting on us to find it again.

In the meantime, we can deliberately "press" these resets consciously in an effort to supercharge the other resets. In doing so, we can truly set our bodies free and enable them to express the movement and the design they were created for.

For example, let's say you are rocking and you feel stuck or tight while you are pushing your bottom back towards your feet. Or maybe you lose your posture and your back starts to round into flexion. If you stop at that point of tightness, or that point right before your back starts to round, you can perform some deliberate diaphragmatic breaths. What you will more than likely find is that your range of motion increases little by little with each exhalation. Your hips will start to open with each breath you take.

You can do the same thing with head nods. If you perform head nods where you feel restricted inside of the rocking motion, you may notice that you sit further and further inside your hips with each head nod. Keep your tongue on the roof of your mouth! It makes your head nods more effective.

For another example, consider rolling, especially upper-body rolling. Imagine you try to perform the upper-body segmental roll and you find it very difficult. Perhaps this is you now. Upper-body rolls are dependent on head control and the reflexive center being "on," Relaxing and performing diaphragmatic breaths could suddenly make rolling much easier. Also, being able to lift the head and drive the body where the head goes, is how upper-body rolling is done. Performing head nods here, may "wake up" the center of your body and allow you to roll with relative ease.

Breathing and head nods can unlock restrictions because they reflexively turn on your center, the middle of you, the "X." Imagine your reflexes are like light switches in a room. If you flip the switches, the lights come on. When all of your reflexive "switches" are flipped on, especially your center "switches," you can move well and express your strength well. You are resilient. Breathing and head nods activate the center "switches," thus allowing you to move the way you were designed to move, keeping your healthy.

This is why these 3 resets are intended to always be running in the background. Your center is always supposed to be "on." That is the key to strength and health: Being reflexively strong from the center.

Do you see the importance of the tongue here? The tongue is also like a switch. When it is flipped "on" in the natural resting position, it encourages the diaphragm to work, and allows the neck to enjoy its full range of motion and maintain its proper postural alignment. This is all crucial to having a reflexively solid center. Therefore, this is all crucial to being healthy and resilient.

The lack of owning these 3 resets is very apparent all around us. Observe people with poor posture and poor mobility. Notice the people around you. Does their head protrude forward? Is their mouth hanging open? Do they have slumped shoulders and tight, rounded thoracic spines? Do they have bellies? It is actually hard to find people who don't fit this description. More than likely the people you observe with these descriptions are all "emergency" breathers, their mouths hang open with their tongues thrust forward—out of its home position, and they lack good head control. Thus, they are weak, stiff, immobile, lethargic, and always tired. They get out of breath easily. They show signs of inefficient metabolisms; and they often have systemic inflammation that is accompanied by aches and pains.

By the way, if this description is you, do not despair. Remember, you can get back to "there." You can restore your body back to the way it was meant to be! Just put your tongue back where it belongs, remember how to breathe, and use your head! This is the foundation. These three things, these 3 "resets," make all the other resets more effective. They can "flip your reflexive switches" to the "on" position and they can help you maintain those reflexes as your standard mode of operation. This removes your restrictions and takes the brakes off your body. They simply restore you.

Make a conscious effort to do these 3 things; especially when you go to press reset with rolling, rocking and crawling. Rolling, rocking and crawling are "good," but tongue position, breathing and head control make them "best." Eventually, with enough conscious practice, these will become subconscious activities that are always "running in the background." When this happens, your foundation will be more solid and you will possess most, in not all, of your original strength.

Say Cheese

When it comes to restoring the Original You, the you that you once were and the you that you were meant to be, it is important that we learn to press reset in all the ways that we once did as a child. There is one reset that we have yet to mention in any book, one reset that you often did as a young child. After breathing properly, this reset could be the most important reset that you ever engage in: Smiling.

Believe it or not, and if you are tracking with this message so far, you might as well believe it, smiling is a reset. Think back to all the images of young children playing that we have referenced in this book, all the images of joy and light emitting from the eyes of a young child. You see the smiles, right?

Children intuitively know, you once knew, that they are supposed to smile. They know that smiling is supposed to be a part of life. They do it freely; they do it consistently. They know smiling makes them feel good; AND it helps them move well.

When we were younger, all of us smiled more than we do today. The cares of this world, the seriousness of our lives, the lull of being sedentary, they have all collectively robbed us of our ability to smile freely. We can choose to smile, and it is a good choice to be sure, but there was a time when we couldn't contain our smiles. They leapt off our faces without effort. What is it that we knew then, but we have forgotten now?

"A merry heart does good, like medicine…"—Proverbs 17:22

Children know this. They exhibit this daily. Adults also know this, and they, too, exhibit this daily, but in reverse. Children smile often, they play often, they move often, and they are full of life. Adults don't smile often. They scowl, they grimace, they frown, they don't play, they don't move; and they feel tired, weary and troubled.

Think about people in your life who are always smiling. How do they move? Do they move well? Do they move often? Have you ever seen

Chris Farley? He was one of my favorite comedians. Chris was a very large man. He should not have been athletic due to his size; or so it would have seemed. However, Chris moved with grace. He was an athlete? Why? He smiled a lot. He had a merry heart—most of the time. Even if he faked it, a fake smile, is still a reset.

Now think about Kevin James, the comedian/actor. He too is a larger sized man who you would not think to be athletic. However, he moves with power and grace. He moves better than most "fit looking" people move. Why? He has a merry heart. He smiles. He laughs.

Jack Black is another larger looking, comedic actor. Remember how well he moved in *Kung Fu Panda*? Okay, that was a joke. But remember how well he moved in *Nacho Libre*? This man is an athlete! Why? He smiles. He has a merry heart.

I use these examples only to highlight that smiling goes together with good movement. It is connected with freedom of movement, with youth and vitality. People who smile often, even larger people like those I just mentioned, move very well. Smiling is a powerful reset. It helps restore, but it also rejuvenates. It keeps you young at heart. And if it keeps you young at heart, it keeps you young at body as well.

Now imagine, do you know someone who always frowns or who is always grumpy? How well do they move? Do they look their age or do they look much older? Do they look tired and haggard? This is the secret that most adults carry around with them. It is the last part of Proverbs 17:22, "…a broken spirit dries the bones." In other words, a life without joy, without smiles, will wear you out.

If this is you, do not fret. There is a button for that. Just smile and press reset.

Again, as children we start out doing things right. We are programmed to move; we are programmed to smile. We were made to have a life full of vitality. This is evident, as it was once written all over our faces.

Just as you have not lost your original movement template, you have not lost the power of your smiles either. You can also dust off your smiles, and rejuvenate your body. Even a faked smile can help soothe your brain and calm your body. Faked smiles still feel good, and they still release "feel good" hormones in the brain.

When we smile, neuropeptides are released in the brain. These neuropeptides help neurons communicate, send messages, throughout the brain and the body.[10] The better our neurons communicate, the better we feel and the better we move.

Smiling also releases neurotransmitters in our brain; dopamine, endorphins, and serotonin are all released by a simple smile.[11] Dopamine is your feel good, reward neurotransmitter. This neurotransmitter may be why people get hooked on drugs like cocaine. Such drugs trigger a large release of dopamine. When you score the game-winning touchdown, or you land that new job, or you simply smile and laugh, dopamine is released. It feels good! Also, it has been discovered that low dopamine levels are associated with diseases like Parkinson's and ADHD (attention deficit hyperactivity disorder).[12] If you remember from *Original Strength*, diseases of the nervous system are also associated with people who skip crawling. Smiling, like crawling, could improve the health of your nervous system. If your nervous system is healthy, your entire body is going to be healthy.

Serotonin is another neurotransmitter that is thought to be responsible for feelings of well being and happiness.[13] It lifts your mood and helps keep you out of the land of depression. Serotonin may also regulate your ability to learn and remember things. If you want to feel good and keep your brain "sharp," smile.

The last neurotransmitter smiling releases is endorphins. Endorphins are the "I am Superman" feeling neurotransmitters. They are natural painkillers and they are responsible for the exhilarating rush people might get from roller coasters or recreational pharmaceutical substances (drugs). Ever hear of the endorphin rush? Endorphins are what can make a man feel ten feet tall and bulletproof. These too, are released when you smile. No wonder children can run full speed into a wall, bounce off of it, giggle, and continue running at full speed. No wonder children

58

always feel so good.

Smiling is a wonder drug. It improves the health of our brain; it lifts our hearts and our emotions. It soothes us; it restores us. Smiling is the movement that is intended to keep you healthy in all areas of your life: mentally, physically and spiritually.

Mentally, smiling helps ward off depression, along with thoughts of anger or fear. It picks us up. Physically, smiling improves the function of our nervous system, which improves the function of our entire body. It improves the way we move and improves our immune system.[14] Smiling also helps us return from the "fight or flight" stage to the "rest and digest" stage. In other words, smiling reduces our stress; it relaxes us and helps us operate optimally much like breathing does when we use our diaphragm. No wonder people who smile often live, on average, 7 years longer than people who don't.

Just like breathing and crawling, smiling is a powerful reset. This one simple movement can change the health of your entire body in an instant. And, because it is a movement, because it requires a thought and an action to carry out, it requires neural connections in your brain to carry out. Just like crawling, the more you smile, the more efficient these connections become. The more efficient these connections become, the easier it becomes to smile and the more powerful smiling becomes. The more you smile, the better you get at it and the more benefits you will reap from it: you will feel younger, happier, stronger, and more resilient.

You truly were made to smile.

The Fear of Freedom

WARNING: THIS CHAPTER MAY MAKE YOU FEEL EXTREMELY UNCOMFORTABLE. YOU MAY ALSO HAVE AN IMMEDIATE DESIRE TO DISMISS EVERYTHING YOU ARE ABOUT TO READ. DO NOT MAKE THIS MISTAKE.

People are uncomfortable with freedom. We make rules to give us direction and guidance. We say cute things like "Rules were made to be broken," but the reality is that we really only say this so that we have a boundary for when we are outside the rules. After all, if there are no rules, how do you know when you have broken them?

This may seem absurd, but we were not meant to be dominated by rules and regulations. Especially the rules and regulations we place on our health. Don't panic. Breathe, and let me explain. If we are truly to return and restore the person we once were, the person we were meant to be, it may be helpful to reflect on how we became that way.

Who taught you how to breathe? Who taught you how to raise your head up so you could see the world when you were placed on your belly? Who taught you how to crawl? No one did. You learned how to move, crawl, and stand on your own, through your own freedom.

Now, who taught you how to eat healthy? Your parents? Your grandparents? How successful were they? When you were five, did you think, "Man, I would sure love a salad," or were you more likely to think, "Yummy! Ice Cream!" It might seem logical, that you should eat the salad. After all, it is full of vitamins, fiber, green things, and other "healthy" stuff. However, in a child's wisdom (yes, wisdom), the ice cream is probably the better choice. Think of all the energy you used to exert: running, laughing and playing all day. Not only that, think of all the energy that is required to fuel a growing body. A growing body that is still running, laughing and playing all day. Which food choice do you think could fuel a body better with such high-energy requirements? A salad, with all its "healthy" attributes, or ice cream, with all its calorically dense fat, carbohydrates and protein? The ice cream wins, hands down.

Ask any child; they will tell you the same thing.

Do you remember, when you were a kid, you naturally liked some foods better than others? You actually chose foods that tasted good, not foods that were "healthy." Those good tasting foods were probably good fuel choices to nourish your growing and developing body. Yet, I am guessing somewhere along the way, your parents fought with you over smashed peas, green beans or butter beans. Believe it or not, you were probably more equipped to make better food decisions as a child than your parents were back then. But I am sure that has changed by now. Somewhere along the way to your adult life, someone introduced you to food rules. They maybe told you things like, "Don't drink milk. Eat your veggies. Eat meat, but not red meat. Don't eat eggs. Eat eggs. Bread is the devil. Don't eat after midnight (Wait, that was the gremlins.) Don't eat after 7:00," etc..

You get the point, right? There are probably more rules about food than there are stars in the sky. And yet many of these rules are born out of confusion. They are condemning in nature, and they are aimed at symptoms in our lives instead of the root causes of our issues. In other words, many of our rules about food exist simply because we are trying to address issues that cannot be solved by what we eat. This creates the need, or opportunity, for more and more dietary rules.

Food is a touchy subject for many people, and it is not the focus of this chapter. I only bring it up in an effort to stretch your brain a little bit in the area of all the rules that surround us. Having said that, let's move on.

Have you ever tried to teach a child how to color inside of the lines? What if that child sees something you can't see. What if that child sees something beyond the lines? What if those lines don't hinder a child's imagination until we teach the child how to "see" inside the lines?

What if all of the rules we create, all the lines we try to color inside of, are nothing more than imagination killers?

From a very early age, the rules of life get piled up on top of us. Some are for our safety, others are "just because." Some rules we somehow choose to ignore, for a while; while others immediately grab our attention and imprison us the first time that we realize them.

For example, I am pretty sure I once got a "frowny face" on one of my kindergarten coloring assignments because I colored outside of the lines. It was a great motivator. I didn't like getting a frowny face from my teacher. She found a way to "encourage" a rule on me and it worked. She motivated me to stay inside of the lines.

When I was in the first grade, my teacher told my mom that I had a hard time staying still in my chair. I did not know this until I heard it. I wanted to please my teacher and my mom, so I learned how to sit still. I didn't want to get in trouble, and I wanted my teacher to like me. Besides, she had a big wooden paddle. Back then, the rod was not spared on children who didn't get in line and follow the rules! The point is, I learned how to sit still in a chair for 6 hours a day, nearly every day because it was expected, and I was becoming a rule follower. I am sure you learned how to do this as well.

As my teacher pointed out to my mom, however, I had a hard time doing this in the beginning. Why? Because my body knew it was supposed to be moving. Sitting still was a rule that was counterintuitive to my design. AND, I did not know I had a hard time sitting still until I heard that I did. I was free to move until I heard that I wasn't. Do you understand what I am saying here? This is a weak example, but a powerful point:

What if all the rules that we create and hold so dear are the very walls and lids that keep us from achieving our full potential? What if it is our "knowledge" of facts, rules and regulations that places limits on our possibilities and robs us of the very freedoms we were meant to have?

Did you know that the more aware you are of something, the more that "awareness" starts to imprison you? Did you ever worry about getting the flu growing up? Did you even know there was a flu season? You know that now though, don't you? Does that knowledge put a slight bit of "fear," or concern in you between the months of November and February? If that is not a good example for you, let me ask you this: Did you naturally become afraid of germs, or did someone teach you to be afraid of germs? Many of us probably licked door knobs growing up, and it probably made us stronger. Fear of getting sick was no concern when you were a child. But today is different. Have you ever shook hands with someone and later found out they had the flu? Did you panic or get worried? Did you feel a "pit of concern" grow inside of your belly? Did you immediately run to wash your hands?

What has happened to us? We live in a phobic world that is caused mostly because of all the information and rules that bombards us. When we were younger, and we didn't know any better, we were amazingly resilient. Rules didn't bind us and knowledge didn't make us anxious.

Today, we have so much worldly knowledge around us, and we have created so many rules to accompany this knowledge, that we have literally lost our freedom and we have become fragile—in both mind and body.

This is not the way it was meant to be. It can't be. We were made to be without limits.

Yes, we do need to practice good hygiene and not all information is harmful. But just remember one thing: It is okay to be carefree and actually enjoy life. It is okay to drop a lollipop on the ground, blow it off and put it back in your mouth. Heck, it is okay to have a lollipop once in a while, too. My point is we need to let go of some things and we need to learn how to be free again.

If you are not sure about this, let me provide some examples I have witnessed:

- I have met people who were physically fine and free to do pretty much whatever they wanted until someone told them that they had a structural issue in their body and they should be careful with the activities they engaged in. This new knowledge put a huge limit in their mind as they now have become concerned that they might injure themselves. Was the knowledge true? Maybe. But when they didn't know any better, they were enjoying their freedom. Now they think they are fragile because someone told

63

them they were. Now, they know they should be careful. They now have "what if..." in their heads when they go to move. What if they were born with this structural issue? Has anything really changed in their body? The only change is the information that they now have in their head.

- I knew a particular gentleman, we will call him Tim, who enjoyed eating most meats until one day he found out all the reasons he shouldn't eat pork. He learned how pigs were dirty scavengers and how they carried horrible bacteria that could poison his body. Do you know what happened? He avoided pork, even at family gatherings where it was the only option of food, even though he was hungry. He avoided bacon for years, even though he lived in the bacon capital of the world and even though he really liked the taste of bacon. The knowledge he gained about pork robbed him of his freedom to enjoy his life at the level that he had previously enjoyed it. Can you imagine a life without bacon? It is a scary thought. Oh, and just In case you are wondering, I am now free from this affliction!

Even though we live in the Information Age, there is a certain level of truth in the statement that ignorance is bliss. We just don't know what we don't know, and many times we are better off not knowing. Many of us would have no limits whatsoever if we didn't know we couldn't do the things we wanted to do.

When we were children we didn't see a set of stairs and think, "They are too high to climb." We simply climbed them. Curiosity begged us to. As children, we didn't have any limits except the boundaries (child safety gates) given to us by our parents. We were creative and we were courageous. We knew how to color outside the lines. And, we knew no limits.

If we really want to regain the person we were meant to be, we have to learn how to unlearn some things. We need to let go of foolish notions like "the body falls apart after you turn 30." We have to learn to ignore and not believe information that is used against us like "arthritis is just a part of life, " or "when you're older, it's harder to lose weight," or "it's natural for your health to decline as you age."

We also have to be comfortable coloring outside of the lines. That is, we have learned that it is okay not to follow the rules when it comes to all the rules that are concerned with the body and how it works. The only rule you should follow is the one that is based off of your design: You were created to move, therefore you should move—often. All other rules, as they relate to how the body works, could probably be done away with if we all moved the way we were designed to move.

Think about it. If your entire life was spent moving and being, much as you did the first five years of your life, the idea of exercise would be a foreign concept to you. All exercise guidelines would be obsolete, or nonexistent, if we simply moved like we were created to move. In fact most of the diseases that we are aware of today would be rarities if we spent our days moving instead of lounging.

We wouldn't have all the crazy rules about nutrition either. We wouldn't have to worry about how many meals we should eat a day, or if we should intermittently fast, or what percentage of carbohydrates we should take in. The rules we impose on our food and our eating habits are mostly aimed at the symptoms caused by not moving the way we were designed to move. These nutritional Band-Aids® would be self-mitigated if we simply returned to the life of movement that we enjoyed as a child. We would be free to eat and enjoy food like we were always intended to. You realize we were intended to enjoy food, right? That is why we have taste buds. Anyway, if we simply moved the way were created to move, obesity would not be an issue, nor would any of the ill health effects that accompany it.

Can you handle the idea that you were not made to follow movement rules and nutritional guidelines? Can you entertain the idea that you were made to enjoy freedom?

You were not born with an owner's manual. No one taught you how to develop and tie yourself together as a child. You followed your own path laid out by your design. Your only rule was to move the way you were created to move. You didn't know what not to do. You didn't worry about what you could not do. You moved where you could, when you could, and how you could. You were free from fears and limitations and rules. You only looked for your potential and you had no self-imposed bounds or regulations. This is the way you were created to be—always.

Your design has not changed. I bring all of this up because when it comes to regaining your original you, you have to be okay with the fact that there is no algorithm. There is no, "if this, then that" sequence. Simply move by exploring the resets, their regressions, their progressions, and do them often. There is no definitive order, there is no concrete set of rules. The only rule you need concern yourself with is engage and move the way you were designed.

Other than that, there simply are no rules.

A New Beginning

Have you ever sat down and thought about the number 40? I know. Why would you? Many of us never give it a second thought unless we are about to turn forty years old. Or maybe we even use it as a "mid-life" number. To be honest, I have never given this number too much thought until my friend, Dan John wrote his book *Easy Strength*.

In the last few years, the significance of the number 40 has continued to run around in my mind. Now, I think I finally know why. Forty is the number of new beginnings.

Let me explain by telling you a few stories that I often heard in church when I was growing up:

In Noah's day, there was a great flood. It rained for 40 days and 40 nights. The world as it was known at the time was forever changed, like an eraser to a white board.

Not too terribly long after that, there was once a guy named Moses. It is said that he spent 40 days on a mountain, fasting and spending time with God. He had received the Ten Commandments! When he came down the mountain, he got angry and smashed the stone tablets that the Ten Commandments were written on! Talk about a "D'uh" moment! Moses then went right back up the mountain and spent 40 days fasting and hanging out with God. When he came down the second time, his face was glowing with the glory of God and the Law was introduced.

Then, there was the issue of the Jews wandering the desert for 40 years before they could enter the Promised Land. The new beginning for the Jews had finally begun.

MUCH later, Jesus spent 40 days in the wilderness fasting and hanging out with God. The Devil tried to tempt Him three times and Jesus sent him packing. Then, Jesus began the process of changing the world.

Not too long after that, it is said that Jesus spent 40 days on the earth after His resurrection. After that, His followers were filled with His spirit and they began a new ministry called Christianity.

And finally, *and I did not learn this from church or the Bible*, a woman is pregnant with her child for about 40 weeks on average. That is, 40 weeks after conception, a new person enters the world. Again, the world is forever changed.

These are just a few examples of how the number 40 has impacted the world for thousands of years. For a good while, I used to think 40 was the number of change. As I was researching some of these stories, I learned that many scholars think that 40 is the number that represents trials. I can understand why some people would think this. All of the above examples do appear to involve some sort of "testing," or non-pleasant experience. However, I think if you really look at these stories and examples I just listed, you will see something a little different. Forty is the number for a new beginning.

Why am I talking about the number 40 and new beginnings?

Because I want you to experience a new beginning. The resets I have mentioned in this book can change your life. They can restore your body and make you "new" again, the new, original you—the you that you once were, made new again. But this newness, this restoration, lies in the consistency of the application. That is why we are looking at the number 40. I want to suggest to you that you "press reset" deliberately and daily for 40 days. I believe in doing so, you will be on your way to experiencing a new beginning.

Can pressing reset for 40 straight days really make a difference in my body even though I'm older than 30?

Absolutely. But you won't know if this is true or not unless you try it. This is almost too simple not to do. All you have to do is spend 10 minutes every day exploring a few of your favorite resets.

By the way, the very first time you do this, you create a change in your brain. That is, you actually create a new neural connection in response to performing a reset for the first time. If you already had that neural connection, you just "dusted it off" and made that connection a little more efficient. The more you press reset, the more efficient those neural connections become at sending and receiving messages. Isn't that awesome? You can actually change the structure of your brain and make your brain better at communicating within itself. Pressing reset also makes the body more efficient at moving, too, because you are actually improving the speed and efficiency from which your brain communicates with your muscles reflexively, thus restoring and improving your reflexive strength.

Remember, your reflexive strength is your original strength, your foundation of strength and mobility. When you possess all of your original strength, your body is as strong and mobile as it was always meant to be. In other words, you are "young" and resilient again.

The challenge is this: Press reset for 40 days, every single day. If you do this for 40 days, you will be different. You will move better. You will feel better. You will be stronger. The best part is, it all starts on day one.

The Forty Day Challenge (These are just examples of what you could do.)

Example 1:

- 10 diaphragmatic breaths
- 10 head nods in the rocking position
- 10 rocks, back and forth
- 10 windshield wiper rolls
- 5 minutes of baby crawling

Example 2:

- 3 minutes of diaphragmatic breathing in various positions.
- 3 minutes of rolling with various rolls.
- 3 minutes of rocking exploring various foot positions.

<u>Example 3:</u>

- 10 head nods while lying on your belly.
- 10 head nods while in the commando rocking position
- 10 head nods while in the rocking position
- 10 rocks in the commando rocking position with the tops of your feet on the floor.
- 10 rocks in the commando rocking position with the balls of your feet on the floor.
- 10 rocks in the regular rocking position with the tops of your feet on the floor.
- 10 rocks in the regular rocking position with the balls of your feet on the floor.
- 5 minutes of backwards baby crawling (keep that head up!)

Again, these are just examples. The resets you need to do are the resets that you need to do. Also, the above examples can all be done in 10 minutes or less. This does not have to be an exhaustive, time-consuming ordeal. In fact, this is probably the simplest and easiest movement restoration template you have ever done (you have already done this once upon a time…). But the benefits will far outweigh any other health restoration program you have ever embarked on. The reason is because you were made to move like this. These resets are how your body was designed to move in order to grow and develop. These movements are already inside of you, waiting to come out to redevelop and restore you; to make you new again.

Ten minutes a day for 40 days = a new you. Can you do this? You have nothing to lose and everything to gain.

Again, Start Where You Are

I have just listed about 40 different resets, or regressions and progressions to resets.

Where do you start? Which resets do you need to embark on?

You simply just need to start where you are. What resets can you do? If you cannot perform the baseline comfortably, simply try the regressions below it. Find the regression that you can perform. Find the regression that is at your limit—you can do it, but maybe it challenges you a little. Play with that regression and the ones below it. Eventually, you will unlock new territory and the resets that where once a challenge for you will become easy. Your body will remember how to perform these movements because they are already programmed into you.

What if you can't perform any of the regressions like you think you should be able to?

Simply regress the regressions. Do what you can do, and start where you are at.

All of us bring different bodies to the table. All of us have a different history of movement, incidents, accidents and lifetimes that make our bodies somewhat "unique." We are all a little different, but at the same time, we are all a little similar. If you have spent 50 years breathing with your emergency breathing muscles, it may be harder for you to find your diaphragm than someone who is in high school. That high school student may only be 12 years out from forgetting how to use his diaphragm. He may be able to find the baseline position with just a little practice. You, however, may have to explore the different regressions, or even find a new regression for yourself. Eventually, you will be able to find your diaphragm. Your body does know how to do it. You just have to help it remember.

What if a regression hurts, or I can't move as far as what I see in the pictures keeping that same posture?

Simply move where you can move. If you can only nod your head about 4 inches before you experience pain, then nod your head 3 inches. Nod your head right before the point where pain starts. Move your head within that pain free range. You are still pressing reset, you are still tapping into your bodies preprogrammed movement template. Eventually, you will restore and reset an even larger range of motion and eventually, you may even restore your complete range of motion—pain free.

If you cannot move your body through the range of motion you perceive in the pictures of resets in this book without losing your posture, that is okay. Move your body to the point, or the edge, of where you can maintain that posture. For example, if you are trying to rock back and forth, but your head starts to drop and your spine starts to flex (round), stop right before this happens. Rock back only as far as you can maintain keeping your head up and your back flat. If you feel your lower back start to round, simply rock to the point before this happens.

Do not stress over having diminished ranges of motion or limitations. *These are only temporary.* You can still work and explore your movements inside the ranges that your body will currently allow you to have. If your body gives you an inch, take it. Sooner or later, it will give you a yard (or a meter for you metric fans).

What if I can't crawl for 5 minutes without losing my breath, my posture, my contra-lateral movements, or my mind?

Just breathe and relax. This is not a pass/fail event. There is no stress here. Your only goal should be to restore your body and become who you were meant to be. Simply do what you can do. Just do what you can do consistently. If you can only crawl for 1 minute, great! Crawl for 1 minute. If your goal is to crawl for five minutes, crawl for 1 minute, recover as long as you need to, and crawl again as long as you can until you can't do it well. Then rest and recover. You can add up the total time it takes you to crawl until you hit your five minutes. OR, tomorrow maybe you crawl for a minute and fifteen seconds. It doesn't matter how you do it. It only matters that you do it.

Just remember that your body already knows how to do these things. You are simply helping it to remember. Don't assume any stress or failures on your ability to do any of these resets. You've more than likely already expertly performed them a long time ago when you were a child. You didn't condemn yourself on your ability to do them then, and you don't need to condemn yourself on your ability to do them now. All you need to know is that you can do them, AND you will do them.

Do you remember the first time your learned how to roll over? Of course you don't. You were maybe a few months old. However, the first time you did it, it was an accident. AND, it was not a graceful looking accident either. You simply, accidentally, discovered you could roll over. Then, you practiced it on purpose. Daily. You also didn't learn how to crawl in a day, and it wasn't graceful the day you did learn how to crawl either. You learned how to crawl by adding several small movements and several small attempts together. And not one time did you condemn yourself or feel like a failure when you were learning how to do this. You joyfully explored and learned how to move through your curiosity and your determination. You did it patiently, consistently, and freely. You learned how to move the right way. You learned how to move by taking what your body would give you. This is exactly how you should go about learning, remembering, how to move again. Explore and take what your body will give you. Patiently and consistently move where you can within these resets. Your body will remember how to do this. It is okay if it looks like an accident the first few times, or even the first few days, that you try to press reset.

It may not be graceful or easy now, but it will be soon. Very soon. Remember how to move the exact same way you did as a child. You were free—free from stress, free from self-condemnation, free from worry. Life was full of wonder and so were you.

You built the perfect body once. Rebuild it the exact same way you did then: through wonder and joyful exploration. Be free and start where you are.

And remember, this is not a pass/fail event. This is your journey, your story. This is only a "pass" event.

Change the way you see things. If your child misspelled a word in a spelling bee, would you say, "You loser. You can't spell anything. You're a failure." No, you wouldn't. What would you say? Maybe something like, "That's okay, honey. You did a great job. You spelled 5 really hard words. You'll be able to spell that word next time." We nurture and build up our children. We know that their "misses" do not determine their worth. Yet, as adults, we forget this when it comes to our own lives. We focus on the negatives, and we allow our few short falls to determine how we see everything. We turn our "misses" into catastrophic, life defining events.

What am I talking about? I once heard a client say, "Man, I've eaten good all week and yesterday I blew it." What she was saying was, "I'm a failure. My one bad meal ruined all my efforts and wiped away all the good I've done this week." She was basically willing to throw away six "good" days for one "bad" day. Truth be known, it was probably only one "bad" meal, whatever that is.

Let's take this further down the thought continuum road. What if she was able to do this every single week? Six "good" days, and one "bad" day. There are 52 weeks in a year. She would basically be willing to throw away 316 "good" days for 52 "bad" days. Do you see what I'm saying? 316 awesome successes tossed away because of 52 misses. Put 316 pounds on one side of a balancing scale and then put 52 pounds on the other side of a balancing scale. Which way do you think the scale will tip? Will it barely tip to the side with 316 pounds, or will it drop with a thud?

This doesn't make any sense. We focus on the wrong things and we turn everything into a pass/fail event. Six "good" days in a week should be celebrated. Heck, four "good" days in a week should be celebrated. For some of us, one "good" day in a week should be celebrated. Our misses do not define who we are. They are just opportunities to learn and grow. They in no way mean we are failures. Yet, we often allow ourselves to throw away our successes over a few misses.

When it comes to restoring the body you were meant to have, focus on the positives. It is pass, not fail.

Just Be

If you have read any of the *Original Strength* books, you know that you were wonderfully made. You were not meant to be fragile or broken. You were made to be strong, healthy and whole.

It is the truth. You were made to be whole—strong, resilient, joyful, alive and free. Just as you were not made to be fragile, you weren't made to be depressed, anxious, fearful and stressed out either. You were made for joy, love and light. You were made to be.

Before I lose you, think about this: Have you ever seen a baby's face when its mother is holding it in her arms and the baby is looking over her shoulder at you? Do you remember any child's face that is exploring your face? What do you see in your mind's eye? Do you see an angry, pissed off child, peering to make eye contact with you? Or, do you see a child whose eyes are full of light, full of joy and wonder? You see the child with their eyes full of life, don't you? And what does it make you want to do? It makes you want to smile back at the child. Their light is rubbing off on you, perhaps? Or, maybe their light is igniting the light inside of you???

Now, imagine a child learning how to roll and crawl. What do you see? Do you see a child full of fear and worry as they try to move across the room? No. You see a child full of joyful curiosity. You see a child whose face cannot help but light up a room. You see a child who is free and innocent. There was a time in your life when you explored the world with this same joyful, wonderful light in your eyes. It was in you. It is still in you somewhere.

Now imagine one last thing: Imagine children skipping. What do you imagine their faces to look like? Do you see a bunch of angry, sad, anxious faces? No you don't. You see smiles. I'll bet you even hear laughter and giggles. Skipping is a joyful movement. You will never see an angry, sour person skipping around.

What is my point?

I have three points, really:

1. Movement is connected with Joy. It brings out the joy and life inside of a child.
2. You were created to move.
3. You were created to be joyful—full of light, energy, smiles and giggles just like you once were.

We have forgotten more than just how to move. We have forgotten how to be filled with joy. Joy, or whatever you want to call it—happiness, light, wonder, excitement, was once a huge part of who we were as developing children. It was naturally in us. For some of us, maybe it didn't last long. But for all of us, no matter how brief it was, it was there. It was in us. It still is somewhere inside.

If you don't believe me, go for a skip. Seriously, go outside, or find a hallway, and skip. I'll bet you can't do it without joy trying to creep up inside of you. I'll bet if you go skip for several yards, you might actually want to smile. It is in you.

In the same way that you were made to move, you were made to laugh. You were made to smile, to have a spark in your eyes. And, your joy, this spark, is tied to the way you move. Again, think of an angry person. Now think of how they move. Now, imagine how a happy person moves. Can you see the difference?

Many of us have forgotten how to be the way we were created to be. We have put away too many things. We've put away much of who we once were. Everything about us is tied to the way we move. It is through movement that we build our bodies, our brains and our emotions. Our "wholeness" is dependent on our design. Our design is largely dependent on our movement.

You intuitively know this to be true. Ever feel stressed and decide to take a walk? Did it make you feel better. Ever get in an argument with your spouse and take a brisk walk, or maybe even run? Did it calm you down? Ever try to combat depression with going outside and taking a walk? Movement is your cure for your "issues." You know this, but you don't know what you know.

We were simply made to *be*. To be in the moment, to be free from worry, free from anger and stress. To be free to enjoy life and all it's wonders and adventures. We cannot be who we were made to be if we do not function, *if we do not move*, how we were designed. An airplane would make a terrible car. Planes are made for the air and not the highway. They have a specific design for which they were created. You could actually try to drive them on the highway, but it wouldn't work out well for long. The plane would eventually wear out and become broken. To use a plane for something other than flying would be ridiculous and even unfortunate.

You, too, have a specific design for which you were created. Look at all the movement capability you were created to have and ask yourself if you were intended for movement exploration, or the still, stagnant life of a chair. You could actually spend all of your time sedentary and live your life in a chair, but your body would eventually break down and become fragile. Why? Because much like the example of the airplane, to use your body for something other than it is designed would also be ridiculous, unfortunate and sad.

Are you whole? Or, are you sad, are you angry, depressed, anxious, afraid or worried? Are you living out your intended design? Or are you trying to live a life that you were not created for? Your life, your joy, your light, is in you somewhere. If you can remember how to move, chances are you can remember how to be.

Strength, health, resiliency, happiness, joy, freedom, mobility and excitement are not independent qualities of one another. They are integrated qualities that all feed and nourish one another within you. They are sums of the whole. The *whole* you. They are in you. Nourish these qualities. Wake them up. Dust them off. Reset your body, Reset your life.

Be who you once were.

Be who you were created to be.

Start Where You Are.

Be.

Is There More?

For me there is. This final chapter is for those who sense there is still more and are seeking. If you decide to read this chapter, I ask that you simply keep an open mind. Regardless of what you believe, the information in this book, and all my books for that matter, will help you restore the body you were born to have. However, for some of you, the information in this chapter will be the most helpful because none of the information I have presented to date is complete without this final part.

And, regardless of what you believe, the only reason you are reading this book is because of a simple prayer. In 2010, I was frustrated. I was tired of chasing my "issues" of pain and weakness, and I was tired of feeling like I was less than resilient. One night, in a hope and a sense that there was more, in a frustration that was fighting thoughts of brokenness, I asked God to show me the best way to train to be resilient. I wanted to be bulletproof.

It was a simple, brief prayer. God took me seriously and answered it. Within weeks, he showed me the heart of what you now know as *Original Strength*. He connected all the dots. He brought it all together. I cannot take any credit for it. Many people that have read *Original Strength* have told me that they can sense my spirituality in my writings. What they really sense is Him.

I am able to write this today because God answered my prayer. He taught me how to regain my Original Strength—All of it. It has been an interesting adventure since I prayed that prayer and I have learned a great deal. The biggest thing I have learned and experienced is that God never stopped answering my prayer. He has shown me, and is still showing me, the true secret to having original strength: It is Him.

If this is too much for you, or if this goes against your beliefs, you don't have to read any further. Please know, if you do not believe what I believe, I still appreciate you and I want you to have the body you were created for. You are not supposed to be broken! The information in this book will work for you and help you regain the body you were meant to have. Please take it and use it. You can regain and rebuild a healthy, resilient body, no matter what condition you are in today.

If, however, you want to know more about what I have learned, buckle up and keep reading.

Original Strength comes from God. He is the source. He created you and you are perfect in His eyes. Understand, I am not talking about religion here. I am talking about The Creator who made you and knew you before you were. I am talking about The Father who loves you. Religion is created by man. God wants relationship with us, not religion. There is a difference.

Anyway, The One who created you made you to be strong, healthy, and resilient in ALL areas of your life. Your original strength is not just a physical quality. To truly be bulletproof and strong you must also be resilient mentally and spiritually. You must have access to a strength beyond yourself.

It is one thing to be physically resilient. It is a whole other thing to be mentally resilient as well. And yet, it is even another thing to be spiritually resilient. In this world, you really need all three to be truly resilient, to be truly bulletproof. It is probably impossible to be physically resilient if your mind is tormented with fearful thoughts of dread and stress, or the cares of this world. If the mind is not resilient, the body will follow whatever condition the mind is in. To truly be physically resilient, a resilient mind is needed. However, how can we have a resilient mind if our faith is weak—if our spirit is weak? We can't. We need to be spiritually resilient in order to become truly resilient, in order to become as originally strong as we were intended to be.

God is the source of all things, especially spiritual resilience. What is spiritual resilience? It is knowing who you are in God's eyes. It is knowing God intimately. It is knowing that no matter what happens in this world, no matter what life throws at you, you are in His arms and they are strong enough to hold you. Knowing you are God's child will make you spiritually bulletproof and it will restore your original strength.

Keep an open mind here. I am still not talking about a religion. I am talking about a relationship.

How do you become spiritually bulletproof, or resilient? By simply **believing** in Jesus—That He died for you: for your sins *and* sicknesses and weaknesses, because He loves you. He is Lord. If you confess this and believe this in your heart, you have eternal life. Eternal life is a relationship with God—here, right now, on this earth.

Don't take my word for this, check it out:
Read Romans 10:9-14.
Read John 17:3

Not only that, but if you receive Jesus as your Lord and Savior, you have a brand new, born again, spirit—your spirit is joined with His. The Spirit of God lives in you. In other words, your spirit IS bulletproof! You are filled with His strength, THE original strength.

Having a bulletproof spirit is crucial to truly having original strength. How easy would it be to be mentally bulletproof if you KNEW that the Spirit of God, the power of God, lived in you? Knowing who you are, and Who is in you—Who will not leave you, is powerful. Knowing you are God's lovely, cherished child will give you the mental peace and strength to overcome anything. Knowing that it is God's will for you to be healthy and vibrant, knowing that you can do all things through Jesus—who strengthens you, will change the way you think! Your thought processes will change! As you realize who you truly are in God's eyes, you will become mentally bulletproof.

As you become mentally bulletproof, you restore the peace and original strength your mind was meant to have. Then, it is even easier to become physically bulletproof and restore your true original strength. As the mind thinks, the body will follow. Once you decide in your brain that you are resilient, safe in the arms of God, you will enjoy this life as you were meant to. The body will follow your decision—especially as your actions get in line with your thoughts! The normal aches and "issues" of the body that eventually wear on the mind and erode its resilience become nothing but gnats. Your mind will resist the urge to focus on these gnats and even tell them to go away. They are only distractions and they cannot hurt you—unless you allow them to settle in you. Eventually, as you realize more and more who you are, the aches and "issues" of the body fade away. One day, you suddenly find yourself strong—not filled with your own strength, but a Greater Strength.

Again, what I have written here was in no way meant to offend you, and I hope it has not. I am simply trying to offer what I have experienced and know to be true. All of what I have shared with you, from *Becoming Bulletproof, Original Strength, Original Strength Performance*, this book and this final chapter have all been given to me by God. When He answered my prayer, He **completely** answered my prayer. He has told me and has shown me more than I could have ever imagined.

In a nutshell, here is what you need to know:

Having original strength is simply having, and being in, a relationship with God.

This is not about religion, or religious beliefs. This is about a relationship with God, the One who designed our fearfully and wonderfully made bodies. The One who created us. Think about it for one second: the pure amazing, awesomeness of the human body's design cries out that God is. He is. He is Love. He loves us with a love that—*if we let it*—can help us to overcome any obstacle and repel any bullet or gnat. He is our strength. He is our source for all good things. He wants us to have a relationship with Him. He wants us to become bulletproof, to have our original strength.

You were meant to be strong, filled with The Original Strength. You truly were. There is infinite hope in knowing this. A hope that does not disappoint.

> "Now hope does not disappoint, because the love of God has been poured out in our hearts by the Holy Spirit who was given to us."—Romans 5:5

References

[1]Sally Goddard Blythe, Reflexes, Learning and Behavior (Eugene: Fern Ridge Press, 2005), p. 20, 59.

[2]Carla Hannaford, Smart Moves (Salt Lake City: Great River Books, 2005), p. 38.

[3]Carla Hannaford, Smart Moves (Salt Lake City: Great River Books, 2005), p. 39.

[4]Sally Goddard Blythe, The Well Balanced Child (Stroud: Hawthorne Press, 2005), p. 35.

[5]http://www.healthcommunities.com/foot-anatomy/foot-anatomy-overview.shtml

[6]Norman Doidge, The Brain that Changes Itself (New York: The Penguin Group, 2007), p. xviii.

[7]Carla Hannaford, Smart Moves (Salt Lake City: Great River Books, 2005), p. 134.

[8]Idem.

[9]Carla Hannaford, Smart Moves (Salt Lake City: Great River Books, 2005), p. 135.

[10]http://www.psychologytoday.com/blog/cutting-edge-leadership/201206/there-s-magic-in-your-smile

[11]http://www.psychologytoday.com/blog/cutting-edge-leadership/201206/there-s-magic-in-your-smile

[12]http://en.wikipedia.org/wiki/Dopamine

[13]http://en.wikipedia.org/wiki/Serotonin

[14]http://longevity.about.com/od/lifelongbeauty/tp/smiling.htm

CPSIA information can be obtained at www.ICGtesting.com
Printed in the USA
BVOW03s1139190415

396768BV00016B/614/P